ACUPUNCTURE TECHNIQUES 101

Safety, CNT, and Needling Techniques

By Cat Calhoun, MAcOM, L.Ac.

Cats TCM Notes Press
San Miguel de Allende, Mexico

*For DeLora, a fellow healer
and a great partner on the path.*

ACKNOWLEDGMENTS

No one does anything truly on one's own. I thought myself totally self-sufficient before I dove into the study of Chinese medicine. When that journey began, my eyes opened to the myriads of those who were actively helping me, those who have gone before, and even those who will come long after I'm gone. We are interconnected. You are me, I am you.

I especially want to thank Dr. Linda Yuxia Qiu, my acupuncture techniques professor, an amazing medical Qigong practitioner, and quite possibly a Daoist immortal in disguise. Thank you for subtly pointing the way to "more." Thank you too, to Dr. Xiaotian Shen, one of my favorite clinical supervisors, for the hands-on teaching and cool clinical pearls you dropped for me along the way.

Thank you to Lisa Lapwing, a most awesome practitioner based in Orlando Florida. We studied together, practiced together, we practiced *on* each other in student clinic, and then we became each others' practitioners! Not having Lisa in my daily life is my one giant regret about moving to Mexico.

Thank you to my buds: Donna "Needles" Tatum, Tiffany Chiu Peralez, Vanessa Olsen, Andi Kohn, Mark Hernandez, and Katherine Webster. To Georgie Hoiseth, a kick ass practitioner and fellow computer geek, I thank thee! To Rita Ramirez, I would *not* want to be on this journey without you!

To my patients, whom I learn from every day and who trust me with state of their health, thank you. I love having you in my life.

And to so many more who have loved, supported, and believed in me, I express my gratitude and thanks. May the deity of your choice look favorably upon you all!

Cat Calhoun, MsAcOM, L.Ac

INTRODUCTION

I took my acupuncture techniques class at AOMA Graduate School of Integrative Medicine in Austin Texas more years ago than I care to admit.

My instructor was Dr. Linda Y. Qiu. She is, hands down, one of the most amazing people I have ever met. I won't lie: she scared the bejesus out of me. It's like that when you are in the presence of a great spirit with a tremendous amount of personal power. I'm not even kidding. She is small of stature, but she could probably kill me with a cotton ball.

So this amazing being who had tremendous control of her own Qi taught me acupuncture techniques. She strongly emphasized the Qi transfer aspect treating with needles.

Her lectures raised questions in my mind like:

- What is it we are transferring to patients when we pick up a needle and insert it through their protective barrier and into their body?

- Are we transferring our own stress, anger, cravings or whatever to them, injecting the pathogen of our toxic emotions?

- How much more effective would my treatments be if I could regulate my own Qi, my own Shen?

- How *can* I best regulate my own Qi/Shen? What do I do to make that happen?

The answer to that last question was I "happened" to take an awful lot of Medical Qigong classes. I mean, I took all three of those three credit hour classes multiple times. I don't think a semester passed in my four and a half years of school that I didn't take one. They saved my life and my sanity. And I have no idea how much they shaped how I treat, but I suspect it's been a huge boost in the effectiveness of my herbal and acupuncture treatments.

If you can do it, take Medical Qigong and take it often from a good instructor. If your school doesn't offer it, check out both of these programs. I will swear publicly to a couple of different deities that you won't regret studying this.

- If you are in the New York City area, find Dr. Linda Y. Qiu (yes, *that* Dr. Qiu…see the 2nd paragraph of this introduction). You can study with her yourself. You cannot go wrong with this.
  https://www.nycemed.com/

  This is a link to a publication she wrote on Qigong acupuncture. Check it out too.
  https://www.nycemed.com/uploads/4/0/8/4/40843695/qigong_acupuncture.pdf

- Sheng Zhen Qigong (https://shengzhen.org/)
  I also studied with Master Li Junfeng a great deal. He has an online school for those who don't have Qigong teachers nearby. I also recommend Master Li very highly.

Take care: All Qigong and Qigong teachers are not created equally. This isn't a martial art. This is a way to calm your mind and your Shen and to build and regulate Qi.

Moral to this story: you will find a lot of text that talks about this in this book. If your school offers only technical instruction, it may not emphasize the critical importance of building good Qi into your treatments. Do not be satisfied with this. Seek out more.

This page intentionally left blank.

TABLE OF CONTENTS

This page intentionally left blank.

SECTION 1
Clean Needle Technique in the Clinic

In the United States you must take and pass a Clean Needle Technique (CNT) exam before you can treat in student clinic. This is important for both patient and practitioner safety. Why? Pathogens, that's why. If you want to stay healthy and keep your patients from getting something awful from your acupuncture therapies, this is crucial.

CNT laws are updated pretty often. I took the class and passed the exam in 2007, so it's a pretty good bet that at least a few things have changed. As of this printing, the most recent CNT manual is the 7th edition. You can download that from the link below at this time in history, but you may need to actually purchase a copy. I had to show mine before I was allowed to test. Your mileage may vary.

http://www.ccaom.org/downloads/7th_Edition_Manual_English_June_2017.pdf

Because the exam changes from time to time, I won't go over that. Get the manual and consult your school for the most recent information. My school walked us through the exam several times during class so we could get the hang of it, learn the proper safety procedures, and would be able to pass the test.

You can take the exam just about anywhere. A friend of mine was traveling for spring break and took hers in Denver even though we both went to school in Austin, Texas.

Once you have taken and passed your CNT exam, the Council of Colleges of Acupuncture and Oriental Medicine will send you a certificate stating you passed. You need to keep that. . .

oh, forever. I had to show it before I could treat in clinic, before I could get my license, and even so I could get malpractice and business insurance. When I double licensed in Florida I had to show it yet again.

What I *will* cover in this chapter is enough information to scare the bejesus out of you about blood borne pathogens and the paperwork involved any time there is an accidental needle stick.

There are risks associated with what we do – big ones. And you need to be aware of them before you start wielding the sharp pointy things.

CHAPTER 1
CNT and Blood Borne Disease

For thousands of years of acupuncture techniques have existed without our current standards of CNT, but techniques of cleanliness have always existed. They just change as our level of knowledge and understanding about how disease is spread changes.

Regardless of the times and techniques that match them, the goal is to prevent the transmission of pathogens. Because acupuncture includes treatment of the body with needles, a huge concern is the possible **blood borne transmission of pathogens**. Current clean needle techniques focus on clean skin and disposable needles to prevent the spread of AIDS, hepatitis, and other blood related illnesses.

In the United States, disposable needles both with and without guide tubes are the standard. This may not be true in other countries. In some countries, needles are sturdier than the disposable kind and can be sterilized with an autoclave, with heat, and with a few other procedures and reused.

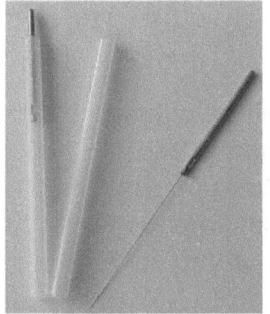 What are those guide tubes I mentioned in the last paragraph? They are plastic tubes cut slightly shorter than the needle that fits into them. You load the needle into the tube, place the guide tube on the skin at the acupuncture site, then tap the needle to get it into the skin. This keeps the shaft of the needle straight, keeps them clean (because your fingers don't touch the shaft that will be inserted) and gives you a quick neat insert into the skin. These tubes were invented by a guild of blind Japanese

acupuncturists to assist with insertion and are now the standard in many parts of the world.

Needles in the US come packaged either in single packs with a guide tube provided for each needle or in multi-packs with 5 or 10 needles per pack and one guide tube provided for each pack. No matter how they are packaged, needles in the US are predominantly of the disposable kind, as are the guide tubes.

In China some practitioners use disposable needles, but many use re-usable needles and use sterilization procedures (like you do for surgical instruments). The needles are used until they are no longer sharp and they are often used without guide tubes. Tubeless insertion takes a lot of practice and finger strength, but does allow for very precise point insertion.

This book focuses upon insertion with tubes, but eventually you will learn some tubeless insertion techniques in your education.

PATHOGENS AND ACUPUNCTURE

There are natural body barriers against exogenous (externally introduced) pathogens such as:
- Intact skin
- Mucous membranes of the nose, throat, urethra, rectum
- Stomach acid
- Healthy cells in nose, lung
- Normal mucus, saliva

These are great barriers, but aren't bullet proof, but of course, you probably know that from exposure to crime shows and *House* and (god help you) *Grey's Anatomy* on television. But there are also an awful lot of ways which aren't so dramatic in which both you and your patients are at risk in your very own office. A few sources of potential infection are:

- Cut skin
- Wounds and microwounds

- Contact transfer
- Hands
- Blood
- Saliva
- Other bodily secretions such as pus or plasma
- Dust
- Clothing
- Hair

Potential infection situations specifically applicable to acupuncture environments can include the following:

Autogenous Infections

In this scenario, the patient is the source of their own infection. They carry the pathogen on their bodies. You, the acupuncturist, can transfer a pathogen from one area of the body to another by reusing a needle.

Moral to the story: don't reuse needles ever, not even on same patient! An example might be a small area of fungal infection like tinea capitis (ringworm on the head) which could be spread to another area by using a needle or other acupuncture instrument (like a plum blossom or seven star needle) on the head and then on another area of the body.

Cross Infections

Patient to practitioner to patient
In this case, the pathogens is acquired by a patient from *another* person or from the environment. This includes blood or secretions from a surface (like an acupuncture table) to your hand and then to next patient. This is a huge uh-oh and the reason we wash our hands compulsively and/or use alcohol scrubs. Hepatitis B Virus (HBV), for instance, can live at room temperature on a surface for up to a week! Holy sick people, Batman!

Blood Borne Pathogens

As mentioned in the example above, blood and fluids (such as sputum, vomit, semen, plasma, etc.) carry pathogens. The most common are Hepatitis B (HBV) and C (HBC). These can be present in the blood or body fluids (whether they containing visible blood or blood in such small amounts you can't see it with your eyeballs).

These can enter through non-intact skin or through mucous membranes. If you pick at your cuticles, bite your fingernails, have cracked skin, have tiny paper cuts, and so forth, your natural skin barrier is compromised and you are at risk. Even micro-wounds you cannot see on your own hands could leave you at risk

Never touch blood or any place there might be blood! Just because you can't see the tiny nicks in the surface of your fingers and hands doesn't mean they aren't there. Patients who have rashes, broken skin and the like are all dangerous for acupuncturists, especially if your fingers and skin areas are not intact!

There is transmission potential for all of the above in this profession because:

- ☯ You are in potential contact with another person's blood or fluids rather often.

- ☯ You are working with various kinds of filiform (solid rather than hollow) needles, which are by design, instruments which puncture the skin.

  It's extremely easy to poke yourself if you're not constantly vigilant. A "needle stick" is when you accidentally poke yourself or someone else with a contaminated needle.

Most often it happens from patient to acupuncturist when you are removing needles. This is why careful practitioners will remove one needle and immediately put it into a proper disposal container before removing the next needle.

Not only is there an awful lot of paperwork if you accidentally experience a needle stick, but there are blood tests for both you and the patient and a whole bunch of worrying about whether you've just exposed yourself to hepatitis, AIDS or some other unknown badness. Not fun.

HEPATITIS AND HIV

These are our own personal Big Bad Wolves. Nobody wants them. They are career and health ending things. No bueno.

When I took the CNT exam, and it seems to still be current, you needed to know the transmission methods, incubation times and several other things about blood borne pathogens. Check the most current manual and with your instructor to get the current scoop.

For now, I'm going to scare you a little!

Hepatitis

Hepatitis comes in an exciting array of colors, all of which will mess you up in various ways. The root of the word 'hepatitis' is 'hepat or hepar, a Greek word referring to the liver. The 'itis' part means inflammation. So this is an inflammation of the liver. If you look back at your Diagnostics[1] texts, you will see that Liver overacts on the Middle Jiao, causing a lot of the digestive problems you see below.

---

[1] Calhoun, *Diagnostic Skills in Chinese Medicine - Book 2: Symptom Analysis and Syndrome Differentiation*, available on Amazon.com in both print and e-book format.

Hepatitis A

Also known as HAV. Hep A is transmitted fecally and orally. It incubates for 15-50 days and then has an abrupt onset. Symptoms include mostly digestive such as abdominal discomfort, poor appetite, nausea, jaundice, fatigue.

It never goes chronic, which is awesome, but it still sucks to get it. There is no vaccine required for this.

Hepatitis B (HBV)

Hep B is a **blood borne pathogen**. This little monster virus can survive for a whole week in dried blood! Talk about a will to live!

The incubation period is long – 50 to 180 days before symptoms show. To make matters worse, the onset is very insidious and gradual. The s/sx are often mild and flu-like at first, gradually progressing to poor appetite, loss of appetite, abdominal pain, joint pains, and rashes. S/sx are often accompanied by chills and diarrhea and last 2 – 6 weeks. After that, the patient often has extreme fatigue and depression for several months.

Here's the really bad part: it can become chronic, so it's a gift that keeps on giving. Some fun facts to know:

- ☯ 5-10% of people who get it get a chronic infection.

- ☯ 30% of all people who get it are *symptom free*! That means you might have a patient with Hep B and they don't even know they have it.

This is why we treat *everyone* as if they have a

dangerous blood borne pathogen and use clean
needle techniques.

◑ 70% recover fully, but are infectious for 3+
months!!

But wait! There's more. After a Hep B infection, liver
cancer is a common thing. How exciting.

There is some good news though:
◑ There's a vaccine for it. It is recommended for
all acupuncturists and needle wielders. Beats the
hell out of possible liver cancer, yo.
◑ The disease responds well to Chinese medical
treatment methods, with the best response from
herbal medicine. Acupuncture helps with stress
levels (high stress makes it worse) and energy
levels.

Hepatitis C (HCV)
Yet another fun blood borne pathogen from the Hepatitis
family, this one incubates 20-90 days and also has
insidious/gradual onset. Symptoms are lack of appetite
(often called anorexia in medical texts), nausea,
vomiting, and jaundice.

This has a strong potential for becoming chronic, which
about 50% of patients acquiring chronic HVC. This one
has **no vaccine** available.

Many people who have it don't know they do. Forty to
sixty percent of liver patients have it. As with HBV,
these patients respond well to herbal medicine.

Hepatitis D (HDV)

This is an infection that is concurrent with HBV and doesn't exist without it. Incubation, transmission, and onset are unknown and there is no vaccine.

Hepatitis E (HEV)

This one is rare in the US, but more common in developing nations. Even some parts of developed nations have them – Mexico, China, and India for example.

HEV is transmitted orally and fecally. Incubation is 15-60 days with an abrupt onset of fever, malaise, poor appetite, and jaundice. Fortunately, it does not develop into a chronic stage. There is no vaccine.

HIV

HIV, human immunodeficiency virus, is blood borne and body fluid borne (that includes vaginal and seminal secetions). Incubation is a beast – up to 15 years!

It's onset is insidious and gradual. Some patients may be completely asymptomatic, but can still transmit the virus.

Symptoms: Initial infection can be like mono: 2-4 weeks with flu-like symptoms. Spontaneous resolution of symptoms, some have no symptoms at all. Later: fever, malaise, body aches, wasting (night sweating, weight loss, diarrhea). Complications include HIV encaphalopathy, myelopathy, peripheral neuropathy, dementia with memory loss, apathy, depression, motor dysfunction, death. Open to opportunistic infections and neoplastic disorders. TB, herpes, staph, hepatits are common as well. Pneumonia is a frequent cause of death.

HIV is by nature a chronic disease and does not currently have a vaccine. As of this publication date, rhetoric is still at the "a vaccine may soon be available" stage. But I've been hearing that for almost 20 years, so….

While you can't acquire the virus casually (handshakes, touching, hugging, holding hands, etc.), you can acquire it from exposed wounds, mucus, blood, spit, etc. You may need to wear a mask and gloves for both your safety and the patient's. Fortunately, the risk for acquiring HIV is lower than it is for acquiring HBV. . . well, that's kinda fortunate. .. but not really.

So how do you keep from acquiring these bad and undesireable things? Get any vaccines you can and use your clean needle techniques. Check your CNT manual for the latest and greatest and remember, you can download the 7th edition at CCAOM.[2]

I am going to cover some precautions that still apply, but again, refer to the CNT manual for the best info.

---

[2] http://www.ccaom.org/downloads/7th_Edition_Manual_English_June_2017.pdf

This page intentionally left blank.

Acupuncture Techniques 101 - Chapter 1

CHAPTER 2
Precautions in Clinic

I got the same mom downloads a lot of you did. One of them was "If you can't say something nice, don't say anything at all." My mom took this a step further and suggested that if I can't *think* something nice, I should change my thinking. Sound advice, but it made this part of CNT very hard to accept:

Treat everyone as if they are infected with a blood borne disease.

If you've read the information about Hepatitis and HIV, you know that patients who walk in for treatment, even if they are coming for something relatively benign and non-diseasy such as back strain, could very well be infected with something that could be cross transferred to another patient or could infect you as a practitioner.

UNIVERSAL CLINICAL PRECAUTIONS

1. Treat all blood/body fluids as if they are contaminated. Treat used gloves and needles the same way. Pretend they are contaminated because they just might be. Remember that many patients of some of the above disease are symptom free and may not even know they have a disease. Or they may know and just won't tell you.

2. Wash your hands often!

3. Use PPE (personal protective equipment), in all situations in which you might be at risk for exposure.

Wash your hands before you put them on and after you take them off!

PPE includes:

    a. Your clinic coat

I have to admit it – I hate these things. We used to call them "polyester cages" in student clinic. Now that cotton clinic coats are easier to find I guess I'd call them "cotton cages." But they still protect you like crazy.

They keep blood and fluids and even shed viruses off of your clothing. It's kind of like wearing an apron when you're cooking so you don't get food and grease splattered on your clothing. You don't really want blood, fluids or other pathogens clinging on to your street clothes where you can carry them home with you, ya know? This is why we wear them in clinic, keep them buttoned up, and take them off before we leave clinic.

Many of my colleagues chose to wear scrubs instead, removing them and changing back into street clothes at the end of their clinic shift, then washing the scrubs after each use.

    b. Latex or nitrile gloves

We've covered that – obvious reasons. Most people don't use them for standard needling, but do use them for any bleeding procedure.

    c. Face shields.

These are less common unless you work in a hospital setting or do a lot of bleeding techniques. It's a pretty good bet some of your doctors or dentists use them.

   d. CPR mouth barriers
When you take your CPR class before you go into clinic you'll learn about these. They're cheap and a lot of EMTs and ER workers (anyone who sees patients who just might need CPR actually) keep them close.

   e. Googles
These can keep other people's fluids out of your eyes.

   f. Aprons
More common in laboratory settings

   g. Disposable masks
You'll see this more in flu season, worn by practitioners who have a cold/sore throat, or by people who are healthy but don't want to get sick during flu season!

4. Use of standard sterilization and disinfection measures as well as infectious waste disposal procedures.

5. Get recommended testing.
Health care workers should be tested for TB, HBV, HCV, and HIV infection prior to treating.
   a. Get tested yearly for TB
   b. Get tested every 6 months if you work in inner city clinics with AIDS and drug patients.

What if you get tested and find you are infected -- can you still treat? Maybe. Depends on expert opinions of review panel including your physician. You also must notify your patients if you are infected.

NOTE:
- Always check for tears and defects in your equipment. Remove and replace any that are defective, broken, torn.

- Used needles should always be placed in sharps containers, even in your travel kit (small sharps containers are made just for this purpose).

CNT PROTOCOLS

Always check the most recent CNT manuals for recommended protocols. Anything you find there will override anything I say here!! This is very important.

Now, that said, here are the definitions I learned. **You need to know the most current definitions!**

Term	Definitions
Sterilization	**Destroys** all microbials including viruses.
Contamination	Introduce disease causing agents into/onto previously clean or sterile objects. Includes touching the needle shaft or cleaning hands then touching something else (patient's clothing, your own, your hair, scratching, etc.)
Aseptic technique	Prevents infection during invasive procedure. Example: cleaning with alcohol.
Antiseptic	**Reduces the *density* of microbial beings on living tissues,** particularly on skin of practitioner and patient, but does not eradicate them. Examples: antibacterial gels and alcohol swabs.
Disinfection	**Destroy or reduce number of pathogens** on **inanimate objects** thru the use of bleach, etc.

Clean field	This is a clean surface on which all sterile (still packaged items) and clean items rest. A clean field also includes the acupuncture points and the skin around them which you will be needling.

Basic principles of CNT

Clean techniques include all of the above plus what's in the most recent Clean Needle Technique (CNT) book.

CNT Principle	Discussion
Wash your hands between patients.	It is generally also considered ok to use alcohol hand scrub when you are in an environment in which you cannot wash your hands.
Use sterile needles	That generally means disposable, but you might end up in an environment in which you use sterilized reusable needles.
Establish a clean field	More on that in just a little while.
Wash hands just prior to needle insertion	If you touched anything non-clean/sterile since you washed your hands between patients….and chances are excellent that you did (i.e. adjusted your glasses, touched your nose, scratched an itch, shook someone's hand, used a pen) …wash 'em again. Or use an alcohol scrub.
Isolate used needles	Many practitioners, especially those who have had to do all the damnable paperwork that comes with a needle stick, will remove a needle and immediately put it either into the main sharps container or into a portable one.
Dress and lab coat	☯ Lab coat should always be buttoned. ☯ Avoid large jewelry, jewelry with

	intricate patterns (which traps germs), loose clothing (which tends to drag across the needles you already put in and drags across contaminated areas and then across the clean areas), and anything else floppy that might cross contaminate. Most acu's don't wear jewelry
Personal care	Take care of yourself, balance your life so you are healthy. If you are healthy and preventative and emotions are good, you can be a good doc. Your energy affects your patients! Cat's opinion: This is incredibly hard when you're in school. Takes even more effort to take care of yourself now. Stay sane and healthy even if that means you have to back off of the fast track that most schools try to push you into. Owing $ to the feds sucks big time, but slowing down a little is better than getting out of school quickly, forgetting 75% of what you were supposed to learn, and ending up sick or crazy!
Get tested for the major stuff frequently	Hep B and C, HIV, TB, and other disease that could keep you from treating.

Equipment Recommends

We use a wide variety of stuff that has to be kept clean. We are gear heads. This stuff takes some maintenance. Here are the equipment recommends for some of our 'gear.'

Gear	Recommends
Needles	Use sterile, filiform needles. In the U.S., they should be disposable. It's required in some places and it's definitely required for getting insurance.
	Always check the packaging for
	☯ Expiration date Yes, they have them. The needles don't necessarily expire, but the packaging does. Once the packaging expires, it's likely that dust and moisture will get in which will corrupt the sterility of the needle/s inside.
	☯ Leaks, tears and punctures. Same deal as above.
	☯ Remove needles from the package in such a way that they remain sterile. Your instructor should show you how to do this.
	☯ If you decide to use multi-packs in clinic, you *can* use partial packs for one patient, then carry the remainder to another patient for use as long as you use a new guide tube and keep the integrity of the needles intact. It can be done. Some clinic supervisors will frown on this. If you know you only need a couple of more needles, consider not opening a multi-pack, but use individually wrapped needles instead.

Gear	Recommends
Guide tubes	You need at lease one sterile guide tube for *each patient*. You *can* use a single guide tube with multiple needles as long as each patient has a clean sterile guide tube that hasn't been used on someone else. If you are just in your learning phase and haven't started treating in clinic yet, consider using individually wrapped needles for now. Fun fact: you can buy packs of nothing but guide tubes. That can be a handy thing to have since sometimes you just don't want to kill off a needle because you dropped the guide tube on the floor. When do you need to change tubes? ☯ When you see a new patient ☯ When you drop one on the floor or table ☯ If you accidentally put the tube down on skin that isn't clean or is infected. Don't run the risk of transferring pathogens to another part of the body – change tubes!
Needle trays and gauze	You generally only use these these for sterilizing reusable needles. There's a whole section in the book on this, about labeling, autoclaving, setting them up, etc. And by the way, you may still need to know the times for each method of sterilization as well as temperatures and pressure releasing and all that. Sidebar: I bought 4" needle saucers (Lhasa's term for it) and use them for guide tubes, cotton balls, and other stuff I need to move around with when I treat. I use these because they are stainless steel and don't mind being sterilized.
Plum blossom needles	Technically you should sterilize after each use. In reality, you can buy disposable versions and

Gear	Recommends
	toss them after usage. I had a hybrid version for student clinic in which only the head was disposed of. Seemed like a better thing for the environment.
Cups	Use glass cups. There is a pneumatic kind with a trigger that sucks the air out, but you can't clean those well and ick could very well get stuck in there. Use glass instead. You can actually clean them well. Here's how you do that effectively: ☯ Clean them with soap and water after each use. Wash out any fluid, tissue, blood, oil, etc. ☯ Soak them in a 10% bleach solution. 10% does a better job of killing bacteria and mold than full strength does. Weird but true. Make a new 10% solution daily because it loses strength after 24 hours. ☯ Rinse them in sterile water and dry them afterward. If you have access to an autoclave, wash them with soap and water to clean out any ick, then autoclave them.
Work surfaces	Clean daily with disinfectant
Clean field	☯ Whether you use professional towels or clean paper towels, only touch one side! Pinch the under side and open that way. Lay it down without touching the clean side at all, not even corners! ☯ The clean field is NOT sterile. It can hold sterile wrapped/packaged items, but once the packaging is open, the shaft of the needle cannot touch the clean field! If it does then that needle shaft is no longer sterile.

Gear	Recommends
	☯ When you put the cotton balls on the clean field, don't touch the cotton balls. Open the bag and move them with your fingers from the outside packaging.
	☯ You should have the container of alcohol next to your clean field. It's best if it's the kind with the pump at the top so you can pump the thing with a cotton ball and soak the ball. Just don't let it drip on your clean field 'cuz that'll lose you points on the impending exam and renders your clean field not so clean.

Cleaning with Alcohol

There is some debate about this the acupuncture community so this could or may have changed by the time you read this.

Step 1 – Clean your hands

☯ Wash with soap and water, scrubbing for at least 20 seconds, rinsing under running water for another 20 seconds. Don't forget to scrub under your nails. Dry your hands on a clean paper towel (*not a fabric towel!*) then turn off the water with another clean paper towel. If you have the faucet handles with the "wings," you can use your elbow to turn it off before you dry on a clean paper towel so that your hands are not contaminated.

☯ Go back to your treatment room being careful not to touch door handles with bare hands. Another clean paper towel will keep your hands from being contaminated.

☯ Soak a cotton ball in alcohol or use a pre-packaged alcohol swab. Use one cotton ball or swab per hand.

- o Wipe palm side first and only wipe in one direction – tip downward - from fingertips to palm starting with thumb, moving over to pinkie
- o Wipe dorsal side next, same technique.
- o Wipe between fingers
- o Use new cotton ball or swab as you feel it getting dry. Don't resoak the same cotton ball!

Step 2 – Wipe the acupuncture points you are going to use

- ☯ Soak a cotton ball (or use a pre-packaged alcohol swab)
  - o Wipe the point to be needled.
  - o Wipe only in one direction *or* wipe in a circle, starting at the center and spiraling out.

- ☯ When the cotton ball starts to get dry, toss it and soak another. Do not reuse it!
  - o You can clean several spots with one swab, but as a rule, change cotton balls when you move from one limb to another, and when you move to the trunk.

- ☯ Let the point dry on it's own.
  The longer the alcohol stays on it, the more microbials it will kill. Avoid the temptation to fan it or blow on it! That gets it unclean again!

- ☯ Only needle when the skin has dried!!!

- ☯ If you think you need to palpate after cleaning, clean a larger area…or palpate and clean again.

Needling and Cleanliness

- ☯ Only touch the needle handle. You can manipulate the needle that way.
  - o Multi needle packs:
    - ▪ Open cleanly
    - ▪ Remove guide tube
    - ▪ Remove one needle by handle only, insert needles into tube with the handle going in first and the tip of the needle pointing out.

- ☯ Needle removal:
  - o If it's tight, shake it to loosen or lift/press point.
  - o Remove needle quickly, press with fresh cotton ball to close hole.
  - o When all needles are removed and accounted for you can break down the clean field.

- ☯ Dropped needles
  Put on gloves. Use tweezers or hemostats to retrieve it off of the floor and transfer it to a sharps container.

  If it was an un-used needle, use your hemostats to pick it up. Now drop it into the sharps container. Now clean your hemostats with the 10% bleach solution just like you do for cups (above).

  If it was a used needle you dropped, bummer. You now have to clean that spot. Put on some gloves and get your hemostats to pick the needle up from the floor. Put the needle into the sharps container. Use 10% bleach solution to clean your hemostats. Also use 10% bleach solution to clean the floor where the needle was (which is why it's better not to needle while on carpeted surfaces). Once everything is clean, take off your gloves and dispose of them in a biohazard container.

CHAPTER 3
Applying CNT in Treatment

OK, let's get to the nuts and bolts of what happens in a clinic with good CNT protocols. This is how your world should look too, both for your safety and the safety of your patients.

To establish a clean work area, you need:
- Running clean water
  You must have this to get your hands and equipment clean.

- Liquid soap, not bar soap!
  Bar soap holds pathogens and contaminants.

- Single use disposable towels to dry hands
  Cloth towels are fine for the bathroom, but before you treat a patient you need to have clean disposable single use towels to dry your clean hands.

- All materials that will be applied to patient's skin must be clean.
  This includes your sheets and pillowcases. Use them only once, then put them into the laundry. Many practitioners opt for table paper rather than sheets for this reason. (But as a patient, I seriously hate table paper. As a practitioner I *still* hate table paper. Super wasteful in my opinion.)

- Clean working surfaces at least once per day, as well as when visibly contaminated.

POSITIONING YOUR PATIENT FOR TREATMENT

Once your clinic is set up for the best clean needle technique and safety precautions, you can think about treating patients.

How you position patients on the table depends on their comfort and also on what points and treatment methods you have decided to use. You have a number of options.

Positioning	Description
Supine	Supine is lying on your back, either palms up or hands on the abdomen. Supine positions give you access to most of the head, the face, chest, abdomen, and the anterior and lateral aspects of the limbs. This is the position of choice for many acupuncture treatments.
Prone	Lying face down. Use a face cradle on your treatment table for best comfort. Some people like to rest their arms beside their bodies, some like to put their arms forward with their hands resting on something under their head. Some face cradles come with a hanging padded shelf for this purpose. You can also use a chair with a pillow placed under the face cradle. Prone positions give you access to the back of the head, the occipital area, neck, all regions of the back, and the posterior/lateral aspect of the lower limbs. This is a great position for a back treatment, for treating sciatica, for cupping and guasha, etc.
Lateral Recumbent	Side-lying, in other words. This is a good position (along with about 80 pillows for support) for pregnant patients. Some of my back pain patients also need this type of positioning. This gives you access to a lot of the body – especially the lateral aspects – but can make getting to all of the points a bit challenging. Not to worry.

Positioning	Description
	You don't always have to treat both sides with all points.
Sitting	This can be a good option depending on the patient and the setting. If you need to needle the neck, for instance, and a patient is very muscled in the neck and upper back or if they are overweight, folds and creases will appear when you position them face down and will make it nearly impossible to needle the neck area. Extremely muscley people sometimes have a lot of upper body bulk and positioning a face cradle for them when they are face down can be a challenge.
	Consider getting a massage chair. Patients with stomach/abdominal pain, extreme lower back pain, or strong asthma will appreciate you for this. So will people who feel emotionally vulnerable lying face down. I'm not sure why that is – you're still pinned down and can't move, but it works for them anyway. It allows people to relax in a position that feels good and gives you access to most of the body. Good stuff.

It takes good time management to do a good treatment. Many practitioners like to do treatment both on the front and back in one session. Combining the front mu points and the back shu points in a single treatment is very effective. But you have to get your timing right so you have enough time to do both sides.

My professor, Dr. Linda Qiu, recommended the prone position first, then supine, as it gives people a chance to really relax for the last ½ of the treatment and catch a brief nap.

WASH YOUR HANDS

Now that clinic is ready to go, let's assume you are finished with the patient intake, have made a diagnosis, differentiation, and have your treatment plan ready to go. You've placed your patient on the table. What's next?

Washing your hands: the most important single procedure for prevention of infection in health care setting. There's a right way to do it.

Table 4.25	
Washing	☯ Get your hands wet, then use liquid soap to lather up. Leave the water running. ☯ Wash the entire surface of your hands: between the fingers, around and under the nails, wash all the way up to the wrist or even mid forearm. It is really much easier to do this if you keep your fingernails short and clean. I was taught to wash while singing the US version of the Happy Birthday song. Sing it two times.
Rinsing	☯ Lower your hands to the soap and water drains off of your fingertips as they are rinsed. ☯ Rinse for at least 20 seconds.
Turn off the water	You need to keep your hands clean, so you don't just reach over and turn off the tap. ☯ If you have the type of faucet handles that have "wings" that allow you to turn the water off with your elbow, do that. If not… ☯ Complete your rinse, leave the water running, dry your hands on a clean single-use paper towel, then use a fresh paper towel to turn off the tap.

Dry your hands	Use clean, single-use, disposable paper towels to dry your hands.

Check your CNT manual for the latest and greatest information about hand washing procedures. As usual, *that* information overrides this information.

How do you get back to your treatment room with clean, uncontaminated hands? If you can teleport yourself, great. But most of us can't do that. Again, use a clean paper towel. Use one to open the bathroom door, then use it again to open your treatment room door.

What if you don't have a sink available? Use an alcohol based hand disinfectant or other antiseptic cleanser. But beware betadine based scrubs. Those have allergens in them some people are allergic to.

If your hands are contaminated after washing, clean your fingers, especially the tips, with an alcohol swab, cotton ball soaked in alcohol, alcohol-based hand rub, etc.

That brings up the question: How often *should* you wash your hands?

- Before a treatment

- Immediately before acupuncture procedures

- After your hands come into contact with blood/body fluids or obvious environmental contaminants

- Whenever hands become contaminated during treatment

- Between patients

☯ At the end of a treatment

☯ After removal of PPE

A lot, basically. Protection for you; protection for your patients.

PREPARING THE SITE ON THE SKIN FOR INSERTION OF NEEDLES

Your first step is to check that the skin areas to be treated are free of any cuts, wounds, or diseases. Further, ensure that the part of the body to be treated is clean. It's not uncommon to find evidence of lotions, creams, sunscreen, even tanning stuff. Clean it off.

☯ Use 70% isopropyl alcohol to prep the patient's skin. This is better than the 91%, which dries to fast to be of use in killing germs.

☯ For immunocompromised patients, use something like betadyne (unless the patient is allergic to that, shellfish, or eggs), then use an alcohol swab or benzylconium chloride to prep the site.

☯ Swab the point once in such a way that the swab or cotton ball touches the area only once so as not to re-contaminate the area. This can mean you do a single swipe of the area in one direction only or you can start in the center and spiral out in one direction only.
   o You can use the same swab or cotton ball for points in the same general area
   o Change swabs/cotton balls when you move from one limb to another, or from limb to trunk. Always use a fresh cotton ball /swab for the face.

☯ Allow the prepared spots to completely dry before you start needling.

o   The more the alcohol dries the more germs it obliterates. In case you are interested, alcohol dissolves the lipid barrier that forms the protective cell walls of a bacterium. Additionally, it causes protein denaturation, disrupting the enzymes within the cell that it needs to function. Bye bye bacteria. This protein denaturation process is also pretty deadly for viruses, killing them on contact. Both bacteria and viruses are more vulnerable outside of the host body, so surface attacks are pretty effective.

o   Not only will allowing the alcohol to dry give you the best critter killing ability, it will also be more comfortable for the patient. Have you ever gotten alcohol on a cut? Not a fun sensation.

o   Reduces the possibility of pushing minute amounts of contaminants suspended in the alcohol into the body with the tip of the needle.

Palpating the Points

This is a crucial step in finding the points you are going to needle. Do you have to re-swab the point each time you do this? Do you have to wash before and after this too? No.

☯   It is acceptable CNT procedure to touch the acupuncture point after cleaning the skin, *as long as the hands have not been contaminated.*

☯   If your hands have been contaminated since your last hand washing or alcohol decontamination, you're good. But using a pen, leaning on something with your hand, picking something up off the floor, scratching your nose, etc. are all considered contaminating events.

You know what I do? Something like this:

- Wash my hands, greet my patient, usher them into my treatment room.

- Do the patient intake, get my diagnosis, differentiation, then treatment plan and have the patient lie down on the table. I put on some nice relaxing music.

- I then use an alcohol scrub on my hands and get my clean field and needles ready. I clean my fingertips with a cotton ball soaked in alcohol and palpate the points or channels. I learn vital information like this – if a point feels hollow or squishy it can mean deficiency, if it feels like it is harder than surrounding tissue or peaks up a bit when I slide my finger over it then it could be an excess or blockage, I might find edema, etc.

- I excuse myself and go wash my hands per CNT procedures. (I do this for cleanliness, but also because I hate how alcohol scrubs make my hands feel – except the EO brand, which doesn't dry so sticky).

- I knock on the door and go back in to the treatment room and swab the points I'm going to use. And then I alcohol scrub one more time before I pick up a needle. (Why? Because I know me. I'm not that careful, so I am pretty sure I did something that brought me into contact with contaminants. That could mean my fingertip brushed the door when I knocked, I decided to add another point and have to open the needle box again, I picked up a pen to note what I just did, adjusted the volume on the music, etc.)

- *Now* I can palpate the point I'm going to needle and insert.

Needles

It is critical that shaft of the needle maintains sterility prior to insertion! Here are the precautions:

☯ When opening the needle packet, make sure shaft doesn't touch part of packet that was touched by fingers when opening.

☯ Make sure your bare hands do not come into contact with the needle shaft!

That's not so difficult if you're talking about a 1 cun needle, but when you get into the 1.5, 2.0 or even 5.0 cun needle lengths, that's more difficult. Then you need to support the shaft in a sterile way.

If needle shaft must be supported, use a sterile gauze pad or cotton ball. Remember: anything you touch with fingers is no longer sterile! Use the still-sterile *inside* of the pad.

Guide Tubes

Guide tubes should be sterile at the beginning of each treatment on each patient. It is considered acceptable to use the tube repeatedly on the same patient, but be sure to use a new sterile guide tube for each patient.

When you are using a guide tube (i.e., not needling free hand), drop the needle into the tube *handle* first. Place the guide tube on the clean field between uses. *Don't* put it back into the multi-pack because it's not sterile after you have picked it up.

USING GLOVES

When do you use them? Do you have to have them on continually? No. Use them in these instances:

- ☯ During procedures such as bleeding where there is a greater risk of contact with larger amounts of blood.

- ☯ When working with patients who have open lesions or weeping exudates from their skin. Like shingles patients, for instance. You definitely don't want to come into contact with that fluid!

- ☯ When the practitioner has cuts, abrasions, chapped skin, hang nails, or broken cuticles on his/her hand and the lesions are location in a location where they pose a hazard.

- ☯ When palpating or needling in mouth or genital area. (It's rare to do this – but if you do, the cleaning procedures are the same.)

- ☯ Use gloves for blood work, for HIV patients with open skin or with HIV bleeding symptoms.

Glove Facts

- ☯ Do you have to glove up for routine acupuncture practice? No, you do not. Not unless you are doing bleeding procedures or the conditions above apply.

- ☯ Gloves will not protect you from puncture injuries. Gloves are a barrier only to blood and body fluids, not pointy needle tips. Only proper handling of contaminated needles will protect you from needle stick accidents.

- ☯ Gloves won't work if they aren't intact! Disposable gloves should be replaced as soon as they are contaminated, torn, punctured, or compromised as a functioning barrier.

MANAGING USED INSTRUMENTS AND UH-OH MOMENTS

We have a lot of clinic bling – needles, sharps containers, cups, trays, hemostats, and so much more. And we have to manage and keep all that stuff clean.

Needle Spills and Sharps Containers

Needle spills – accidentally dropping one or more used needles – are bound to happen at some point. Here's what you do about it.

☯ Use gloves and hemostats/tweezers to recover them.

☯ Clean spill area with soap/water

☯ Wipe exposed surfaces with germicide such as bleach (10% bleach solution works).

☯ All materials used in clean-up job (paper towels, etc.) should be discarded with double wrap (and placed into a biohazard container)

☯ Wash your hands!

I've already told you this, but you need to dispose of used needles or sterilize them if you practice in an area where that is the standard. If you are in an area where disposable needles are the norm, strongly consider using small sharps containers you can carry with you as you remove needles. This will seriously reduce the risk of needle spills.

If you do use sharps containers, regardless of size, you need to send those off for disposal when they get ¾ full. Don't cram more needles in there. You're bound to get stuck at some point if you do.

Bleeding During Cupping

Whether your patient bled during cupping unexpectedly or you are intentionally using cupping to help with a bleeding procedure, dealing with blood in a safe manner is important.

Here's what to do when you are dealing with blood and cups. We're assuming in this discussion that the cups have been on for the appropriate length of time and you now need to remove the cups without getting blood everywhere. Cuz who wants to clean up a mini-crime scene?

1. Gather your gloves and cleaning materials.

2. Put on gloves.

3. Remove cups, taking care to prevent fluids from spreading/splashing.
    a. Take the cups off with the first edge pointed away from you.
    b. If there is a lot of blood in the cup, use paper towels on that side to keep it from spilling. Although, that said, blood inside of a cup tends to congeal really quickly, so it's not that big of a challenge.

4. Stop bleeding through the use of appropriate pressure. Paper towels or cottonballs are fine for this.

5. Clean up any bleeding that has occurred. Handle/dispose of all cleaning materials used in a biohazard waste container. I don't use the same one I use for needles – I have a special one for this and

only put the bleeding stuff into it. That's just me.

6. Immediately isolate the cups.
    Sterilize the cups using a double sterilization
    procedure w/chemical disinfectants.
    Read on to find out what double sterilization is.

Note that disposable, plastic or rubber cupping devices that
can't be sterilized should be used on only one patient! And I
mean *dedicated* to that one patient.

You *can* sterilize the silicon cups, but I find I don't get
fantastic suction with those. Nice for use on the face though.
And you can do sliding cupping with them. But I still prefer
the glass.

And by the way? I always point the cups away from me
when I release them. There could be tiny body fluid droplets
in there that spray and I can't see them.

Blood and Body Fluid Spills

We're not talking gallons or even cups of the stuff, but it's
still considered a "spill." I've had to do it a few times. It's
not so bad.

- Wear disposable, waterproof gloves for this

- Clean the spill once with soap and water.

- Wipe all exposed surfaces with a germicide.

- All materials used in the clean-up job should be
  discarded in double wrapping.

- Wash your hands at the end of the cleanup.

There is a standard emergency spill kit that can be acquired easily. I've seen them in hospitals and they are kind of brilliant. They consist of: gloves, a powder you put on blood spills that is fluid controller/solidifier to absorb blood, a scoop for picking up the solidified blood, germicidal disposable wipe that stays in place for a certain number of minutes, hand cleansing wipes, biohazard bag. There also caps, shoe covers, face mask, and gown in this kit. It's a little over the top for a standard acupuncture clinic, but if you happen to do a lot of bleeding procedures, might be worth assembling one.

What if blood or fluid gets onto your nice white clinic sheets?

This isn't on anyone's test, but I think it's good advice.

I only use white clinic sheets. That may seem kind of sterile, but I have reasons. First, it has a "spa" kind of feel. It also looks super clean and legit. Most people perceive white as clean, fresh, and disinfected. A little color psychology for you. You're welcome. Finally, believe it or not, white sheets are actually really easy to get clean after a blood spill because you can use hydrogen peroxide on them to bubble the blood loose and you don't have to worry about a bleached out spot on a colored sheet.

And blood spills happen more often than you might think. Most of the time I see small drops of blood after needle removal. I'm careful and make sure the points aren't bleeding, but sometimes the point doesn't *start* bleeding for a few seconds afterwards. That can leave small drops of blood on a clinic sheet.

And even small drops of blood on a clinic sheet have got to be dealt with quickly. As soon as your patient has left the room, you need to get the blood out of that sheet.

1. Glove it up in disposable waterproof gloves.

2. Remove the sheet and head to the clean up sink. Grab a bottle of hydrogen peroxide on the way.

3. Stretch the affected part of the sheet over the sink and kinda poke it own a bit so that you make a little "bowl" with the bloody dots at the bottom.

4. Put a cap full of hydrogen peroxide on the blood and enjoy watching it bubble for a moment.

5. When it slows or stops, scrub it together a little bit to help break the blood up, then repeat step 4 and then this step.

6. After the 2nd round of hydrogen peroxide and scrubbing, you should see a noticeable difference in the blood stain. If you did it right you will probably see a little bit of yellow. Cool.

    Rinse in running water. Put a little bit of liquid soap on the former blood spot and scrub it together like you did in step 5. Rinse it again and the stain should be gone. If not, a little more soap and water should do it.

If you clean up quickly soon after the spill occurs you will get that puppy clean. Wring it out and hang it somewhere to dry out before you put it into the laundry or it could grow mold.

DISPOSING OF BIOHAZARDOUS WASTE

First, what all is considered biohazardous waste?

- ☯ Any solid waste or liquid waste that may present a threat of infection to humans. That includes:
    - o Discarded sharps (used needles)
    - o Human blood
    - o Clinic waste such as table paper or cotton balls that contain human blood
    - o Body fluids
    - o Non-liquid human tissue and body parts
    - o Human blood products
    - o Laboratory disease-causing agents

Biohazardous waste, except for sharps, must be packaged in impermeable, red, polyethylene or polypropylene bags, and sealed.

Discarded sharps must be separated from all other waste and placed in leak-resistant, rigid, puncture-resistant containers. In most communities that means the red sharps containers you get from biohazard suppliers, but there are some communities that allow sharps to be placed in any leak-resistant, rigid, puncture resistant containers as long as they are properly labeled. Some places require the lids to be glued shut.

Regardless of type, all biohazard containers have to be clearly marked.

What do you do with the containers now that you have them? When they are full to their designed capacity, you call a biohazard company to come pick them up. Some manufacturers will provide free return shipping and shipping return boxes in the cost of the container, which is awesome. That's my favorite way to deal with biohazardous waste. Seal it up as per their instructions, ship it back.

You might also see big boxes with what look like red trashcan liners in your student clinic. As student interns, we were allowed to put our filled sharps containers into these boxes. You can get this same arrangement on a smaller scale when you get your license and have your own clinic.

WORKING IN PUBLIC HEALTH CLINICS

Public health settings include detox clinics, stop-smoking clinics, AIDS clinics, TB clinics, and institutions such as jails, public hospitals, and community centers.

Characteristics of public health clinics vary, but often include:
- ☯ Have group treatment rooms where several clients sit and receive ear or body acupuncture.

- ☯ Many of those rooms do not have sinks in them. So you have to use a lot of alcohol based hands scrubs and plan for hygiene that doesn't involve running water.

- ☯ Many of these settings target troubled populations such as drug and/or alcohol addicts. You could find a lot of peopled who have concurrent HIV, hepatitis, tuberculosis, mental illness, homelessness, malnutrition, poverty and more. These folks frequently have a long history of illness and debilitated immune systems.

So that 2nd item up there? That is one of several considerations to think about when working in a public health setting. Here are some more.

Special CNT Requirements for Public Health Settings

It's often hard or impossible to wash your hands as frequently as you do in a private clinic setting. How do you handle that? Like this:
- ☯ Wash hands with soap and water before and after work shifts

- ☯ Wash hands with soap and water (if possible) or alcohol based/germicidal hand rub immediately prior to performing any acupuncture
- ☯ Wash hands with soap and water between treatments as often as possible. An alcohol based hand rub, antiseptic towelette or germicidal hand scrub should be used provided that only the needles, sterile packages and other materials needed for treatment were touched.
- ☯ Wash hands immediately with soap and water after contact with blood or a break in the clean field between or during treatment.
- ☯ Wear gloves when there is a biohazard spill.

Choice of instruments

If at all possible, use disposable, single use needles!

Positioning the patient

Many times your only position option in public health settings is sitting in a chair. Make your patients as comfortable as possible.

This obviously means you can't do stuff you do in student clinic or in a private clinic setting – like needling directly on the sciatica points, lower back, chest and abdomen, etc. This also limits your options for cupping and gua sha.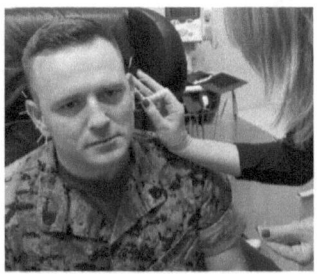

Make it a goal to learn auricular acupuncture and distal needling methods such as Master Tung or Tan's Balance Method so that you can treat absolutely anything using points from the elbows and knees down, ears, and head.

Removing needles

- It is critical to carry an impervious sharps container so that the needles can be disposed of immediately. That probably means you'll be using the small pint sized containers.

- Count the needles you've used and count the ones you remove to make sure it matches! Note this in the patient chart!

- Check chairs and surrounding areas for fallen needles before, during and after each session. I find it helps to use the flashlight app on your phone or carry a small flashlight to spot them. I shine the light at floor level and can see the gleam easier that way.

- Instruct clients *not* to handle needles if the needles fall out or if they fall after removing them. People want to be helpful most of the time, but ask them politely not to and hope for the best. They'll probably do it anyway.

  By the way, this is a likely place for needles to fall out. People are awake, maybe interacting, reading magazines, moving more than they would if they were lying on a table.

- Check for bleeding that may have occurred at the needle sites. Also watch for *delayed* bleeding afterwards and check for small areas where the needles were that are puffing up and looking a little blue. That's a bleeder under the skin. It generally stops quickly on its' own, but can leave a bruise, so I apply medium pressure to these sites with a cotton ball until I feel sure it's stopped bleeding. I explain what happened and ask the patient to rub it gently to help the blood under the skin disperse.

> There's a much higher risk of needle sticks and needle spills in a public health settings. Take extra care!

The NADA Protocol

This is used a lot in public health settings. These are a series of bilateral points on the ears that help detoxify the body of chemical substances (tobacco, alcohol, drugs) and help calm the mind and cravings. These points focus on the three organs that are responsible for removing toxic chemicals from the body – the lungs, kidney, and liver.

This is an excellent protocol to know and practice. Always check to see if those points are bleeding after you remove the needles. These are very shallow spots with a ton of tiny blood vessels in 'em so they tend to bleed easily. Use a cotton ball and press for several seconds until the bleeding stops. Don't forget your precautions about blood. It probably won't bleed a lot, but if so, snap on a glove before you press with the cotton ball or paper towel.

Cat's tip: Carry Q-tips in a ziplock bag in your kit. Use these instead of cotton balls on ear bleeds. Lot's easier to get to the bleeding spots and apply a little pressure to help them quit bleeding.

CHAPTER 4
Sterilizing Instruments

This is important stuff if you are taking the written portion of the CNT exam. You need to know it cold. You also need to memorize **the most current material from the most current version of the CNT manual.** Don't rely on this information. I took these notes some time ago.

And by the way, for those of you who do use re-useable needles:

1. Put them into a disinfectant solution immediately after use.
2. Remove the needle/s from the disinfectant while wearing gloves and using tweezers or hemostats to pick up the needle, then soak in water to loosen any materials that might remain.
3. Check the needle for damage, burrs, etc (using cotton –drag needle across cottonball). Discard all defective needles!
4. Prep a needle tray w/gauze, needles sticking up
5. Autoclave it

APPROPRIATE METHODS OF STERILIZATION
Sterilizing is the elimination of *ALL* microbial life on an inanimate object! Boiling water, alcohol and pressure cookers don't do the trick—they reduce, but don't eliminate.

In clinic, this applies to those of you who live in an area where needles are re-used. If you use disposable needles, you might still need to know this for any sterilizable equipment you have.

Regardless, you still need to know it for CNT exams.

Autoclave

- ☯ 250°F (121.1°C), 15 lbs of pressure for 30 minutes
  The pressure *must* be released quickly at the end of the
  sterilization cycle. It is the sudden drop in pressure that
  breaks down cell walls of resistant spores. This is
  essential to the sterilization process.
- ☯ If equipment is submerged in water being heated under
  pressure, is does *not get sterilized*!
- ☯ Neither do needles that are lying on a tray in the
  autoclave. At least one side didn't get sterilized in that
  scenario.

Dry heat

- ☯ 2 hours, at 338°F (170°C)
  Dry sterilizers use higher heat and require longer times
  due to lack of pressure release at the end of the
  procedure.

Chemical sporicides sterilant

I don't have much to say about this other than "hey, that's
another method." Also, chemicals. Ick.

Ethylene oxide

Same comments as directly above.

UNACCEPTABLE METHODS OF STERILIZATION

Boiling water

No. That only works in old Hollywood movies.

Alcohol

Alcohol will *disinfect* but will not sterilize. That's why you
see things like 99.9% effective against…. That's not sterile.

Pressure cookers

Nope. Not reliable. Don't.

Chemical disinfectants (not sterilization agents) are classified as follows. The last row tells you how to label them in the clinic.

CDCP	❧ High level disinfectants ❧ Intermediate level ❧ Low level
EPA	❧ Sporicides ❧ General disinfectants ❧ Hospital disinfectants ❧ Sanitizers
Types of disinfectants	❧ Dilutions of sodium hypochlorite (household bleach) solutions ❧ Lysol: intermediate or low-level disinfectant ❧ 70% alcohol: intermediate-level disinfectant
How do you label your disinfectants?	Label should include: ❧ What the solution is ❧ When it was mixed ❧ Concentration Example: 10% bleach, 5/18/2019. And again, 10% bleach solutions (10% bleach, 90% water) work better to kill mold and germs than higher concentrations. Go figure.

In clinic, use bleach, Lysol, or 70% alcohol as a chemical disinfectants.

THE DOUBLE STERILIZATION PROCEDURE

1. Preliminary sterilization
   a. Used needles and other contaminated equipment should have a preliminary sterilization immediately after use, without cleaning or handling in any way.
   b. It is recommended that instruments are soaked in chemical disinfectant for the preliminary sterilization.
   c. Autoclave is not recommended for this step! (Why? If contaminants are on equipment/needle this "cooks on" and still isn't sterile even if autoclaved.)
2. Cleaning and inspection after the first sterilization
   a. Gloves should be worn during this procedure.
   b. Instruments should be soaked in water to loosen any material that may remain, then wiped carefully and rinsed thoroughly. The cleaning itself will not kill infectious agents, but it is necessary to physically remove organic material such as blood or other body tissue prior to the final sterilization.
   c. Inspect the needle to determine if it is defective. (After many uses and sterilization they tend to get bends, pitting, cracking, etc. Drag the needle thru cottonball and see if it catches any of the fibers and you'll know. A needle in good shape will slide right through and won't grab any of the cottonball fibers.)
   d. Discard any defective or damaged needles.
   e. Needles to be reused may be stored and packaged for final sterilization and storage. (You use stainless steel needle trays with lids with a layer of gauze in the bottom. Needles are poked obliquely into gauze pad. The whole needle tray is autoclaved with the lid off or loosened so steam can get to needles and sterilize. You can't autoclave them with the needles laying in the bottom of the

tray because the part touching the tray won't be sterile.)
3. Final Sterilization
    a. Chemical sterilants are not suitable for this procedure!
        (You must use an autoclave or dry heat sterilization method.)

PACKAGING INSTRUMENTS FOR AUTOCLAVE STERILIZATION

Packaging must be judged by 3 criteria
- Is it packaged in such a way that the steam or hot air has full access to each needle and other instruments during sterilization?
- Is all equipment fully protected from contamination once it is removed from sterilizer?
- Can single needles be removed without contaminating the remaining ones?
  (I.e., you have to have enough room to pull the needle out without touching anything else.)

Single-treatment packets are the safest system. That means all of the needles from one patient go onto the tray for sterilization.

Covered trays:
- Needles should be placed obliquely or vertically into a bed of cotton or gauze, in a position that single needles can be removed w/o touching the shaft of a needle or interior of container.
- When tray is put into the sterilizer, the lid must also be placed in such a way that the container *is not sealed*. The steam or dry heat must get to all parts of the needle and any instruments in the autoclave/dry heat sterilizer. Even better is to take the lid off and do a single layer at a time.
- When sterilized material is dry, container should be closed. Tray can then be removed from sterilizer.

☯ Sterilizing needles loose in the bottom of a tray is not acceptable! Not all sides will get sterilized this way.

Label all packages for sterilization
☯ Strongly recommended that all sterilized equipment is marked so as to distinguish it from equipment that has not been sterilized. Use autoclave indicator tape on the exterior of the container.

☯ It is strongly recommended that you use bioindicators when autoclaving instruments so that you know they got sterile. The type that changes color or melts in their tube will help you determine if the pressure and temperature in the autoclave were sufficient for sterilization. This does *not* tell you if the packet was indeed sterilized – just that conditions were right.

CHAPTER 5
Risk Reduction

I should have called this "another way not to get successfully sued." These are some excellent risk reduction notes to help you with that.

OFFICE ENVIRONMENT

Your office environment should be free from obstruction, fall hazards (like clutter, cords across the walkways, bad lighting, etc.)

☯ Lighting
You really need adequate lighting! In the treatment room, use bright enough light so you can see. It's fine to toggle it down to soft lamps after you get the needles. You also need adequate light so people can navigate your environment without tripping on stuff in the dark.

☯ All electric installs should be within local code. Have regular inspection and do any maintenance required.

☯ Keep it Clean!!!
Your clinic space needs to look professional and comfortable. It needs to help your patients relax. *You* need to look secure, confident, professional, welcoming.

Have you heard that saying about serving food, "you eat with your eyes first?" That means that the presentation of the food you serve should look as appealing as possible. The same is true with you and your clinic environment. You start treating a patient as soon as they walk in the door. Make it good. Look around at different acupuncture offices. Make notes about what you feel works and what doesn't.

Informed consent and paperwork

☯ You need patient paperwork for everyone and it needs to be signed and dated. Check out the student clinic consent and paperwork forms in use at your school.

☯ Informed consent paperwork should reflect the procedure that patients are asking to give consent to. This shows that the person consenting understood the nature of the procedure, alternatives, the risks involved and the probable consequences.

☯ HIPPA forms
If you are treating in the US, this is crucial.

☯ Any other medical records
Sometimes patients bring medical records from other docs. This goes in their files.

All paperwork should be filled, signed, and dated *prior to treatment!!!* Don't do *anything* without signed, dated paperwork. Always check the paperwork yourself before you treat. Clearly explain what procedures like gua sha and cupping will do to the skin!

Don't let this be a surprise. Always ask if a patient is going to be going to a formal event or on a honeymoon, anything where they might not want bruising on their skin.

SOAP Notes

This is about maintaining accurate records of patient intake, follow-up, and treatment. You can do this digitally or manually.

"SOAP" notes are how the medical community keeps track of patient complaints, medical history, objective information, assessment, diagnosis, differentiation, and treatment plan for a patient visit.

SOAP stands for Subjective, Objective, Assessment, and Plan. All medical forms follow this basic structure even if it doesn't say these exact words. Let's break it down.

S = Subjective

This is what the *subject*, i.e. your patient, tells you. This includes the Chief Complaint (often abbreviated CC). It also includes the patient's medical history and/or the history of the CC.

O = Objective

This is the information you gather from observation. This includes all of those skills from the first Diagnostics book [3]– observation, palpation, smelling, listening, pulse diagnosis, tongue diagnosis, questioning, etc. It can also include blood pressure and respiration rate and any other medical assessment methods you use.

A = Assessment

This is your assessment of what is going on. It includes the diagnosis and the differentiation.

☯ Diagnosis.

The diagnosis should clearly reflect the CC (chief complaint). Please note that in the United States we are limited to a certain range of diagnoses! We can say "lumbar pain" as a diagnosis, but we can't say "herniated disc," as this is outside of our scope of practice. Check with your clinic supervisor for a list of allowable diagnoses. In the US this is a range of the ICD

---

[3] Calhoun, *Diagnostic Skills in Chinese Medicine Book 1: The Four Diagnostic Skills* (ISBN 1097891062). Available on Amazon.com in both digital and print formats.

codes that are used for coalescing a diagnosis down to an alpha-numeric code so that it's easier for insurance to bill...and often to deny payment for treatment. Just being real. I hate dealing with insurance.

☯ Differentiation
Differentiation is *why* the diagnosis exists. This comes from all of the cool listening, smelling, asking questions, etc. skills you have. Let's use a diagnosis of "Left side lumbar pain" as an example. The differentiation is what is continuing to cause that. Here are some possible differentiations:

☯ Qi and blood stagnation
☯ Kidney Qi deficiency
☯ Blockage in the Dai channel

> Can you say "due to disc herniation?" No, you cannot! We have no way of verifying that and it's outside of our scope of practice.

> Can you use more than one TCM type differentiation? You may indeed. In the above example a patient can be suffering from Qi and blood stagnation stemming from Kidney Qi deficiency, so yes, you can use more than one.

P = Plan
Once you have your assessment, this gives you a pretty good idea of what you need to do.

The Plan section details what points you will use, what sides of the body those points are deployed on, other treatment methods (like cupping, e-stim, gua sha, etc.), and herbal formulas you are prescribing.

It also includes instructions to patient and the number of needles you used and disposed of.

Your records should give a very accurate picture of what was done in the clinic, what treatments are working, and what didn't.

This is very important. Burn it into your brain:

Any of your patient records can be subpoenaed at any time. Always write your records as if they are going to be!

Daily Appointment Schedules

Records of daily appointment schedules must be *retained*! This is critical, especially for public health concerns. It's the law in the United States.

PATIENT CONFIDENTIALITY

Practitioners may not release any information in the United States without *written* patient consent! Verbal just doesn't cut it, peeps.

You may discuss cases with others, but *without* any identifying information of any kind. If you give out enough information that someone could easily identify someone ("Oh, that must be Brad from the 2nd floor."), then you've just violated HIPPA. And that's an expensive violation, lemme tell you. It's a bad idea to discuss patient cases with people who aren't medical personnel. It's not a source of entertainment; it's people's lives. They may not want you discussing their health issues with anyone else. While not explicitly illegal, it's just a bad idea. Especially in a public setting.

And while we are on this topic, if you see a patient in public, don't approach them to offer a hello. Maybe they don't want people knowing they are going to anyone for treatment and your casual greeting could raise awkward questions for you. If they approach you first, then you're fine. Just don't initiate it yourself. If they ask you about it the next time they come in for treatment – like "hey, why didn't you come say hi" – then you can say that you didn't know what their comfort level was with having to explain that you were going to someone for acupuncture, so you wanted to give them space.

No one has ever had this conversation with me. Usually it's the opposite. The last one I had like this was after seeing a fertility patient and her mom at a coffee shop. It was more along the lines of 'Oh, thank you for not outing me! I didn't know how to explain how I knew you and I don't want my mom knowing I was coming to your for fertility treatments because I'm just not ready to have that conversation yet!'

If you are part of a healing team this changes of course. Some groups of acupuncturists who work together will debrief at the end of the day or week and discuss patient cases. That's fine since all personnel who legally work for an acupuncture clinic are bound by the same confidentiality laws.

Medical practitioners, including acupuncturists are considered to be **mandatory reporters**. This means we are bound by law to report known or suspected communicable diseases that are a risk to public health (like tuberculosis for instance), child abuse, and elder abuse. In some areas you must also report suspected spousal abuse. Check the laws in your area.

You *can* discuss cases for underage patients (17 years or younger) with parents as long as they have at least partial custody of the minor. After this person reaches the age of 18, you can no longer discuss their case with their parents without their written consent.

In general:

☯ You must have an OSHA Blood Borne Pathogen and Exposure Control Plan on file and everyone you work with or who works for you must know where it is and how to access it and be familiar with it.

☯ Treat all blood and body fluids as if they are contaminated.

☯ Wash your hands per CNT protocol

☯ Use gloves and PPE as required

☯ Use standard sterilization and disinfection methods.

☯ If you work in an are where there is a likelihood of exposure, you should *never*:

☯ Eat, drink, smoke, apply cosmetics, or apply lip balm

☯ Handle your contact lenses.

☯ Keep food or drink in refrigerators, freezers, shelves, cabinets, or countertops where blood or potentially infectious materials might be kept.

What to do in the event of exposure

☯ Contact on skin
In the event of unexpected contact with fluids/blood or if no gloves are available, wash your hands and other affected skin with soap and water for at least 10 seconds after the direct contact has terminated.

☯ Contact on mucus membranes
In the event of blood/fluids coming into contact with mucous membranes (in your nose, mouth, eyes, etc.),

flush with running water 15 minutes minimum!

☯ Report it.
If you work for someone else or are an intern in student clinic, report all exposures to your supervisor as soon as possible. Fill out an exposure report form and get post-exposure medical evaluation and follow up as soon as possible.

Ask the patient to do likewise. They may refuse. You can't control that.

Keep records of this for yourself - this should include your current HBV vaccination status, post exposure evaluation and follow-up information. Also note any results from the patient and whether they refused the post exposure evaluation.

☯ Decontaminate.
You need to decontaminate all surfaces, tools, and equipment that were exposed to blood or other potentially infectious materials. These must be decontaminated and sterilized as soon as possible before servicing or being put back to use.

You should decontaminate by using: Decontamination
   o A solution of 5.25% sodium hypochlorite (household bleach) diluted to between 1:10 and 1:100 with water.
   o Lysol or other EPA-registered tuberculocidal disinfectant.

☯ When cleaning up a spill of blood, carefully cover the spill with paper towels, then gently pour the 10% solution of bleach over it, and leave it for at least 10 minutes.

- When decontaminating equipment or other objects (tweezers, first aid boxes, you clinic box, etc.), leave the disinfectant in place for at least 10 minutes before continuing the cleaning process.

NEEDLESTICKS AND ACCIDENTS

> The risk of infection from a needle stick:
> HBV: 6-30%
> HIV: 0.5% [4]

In the United States, OSHA requires that the HBV vaccine must be available for all employees who have occupational exposure. If you run a clinic, you have to offer this.

Further, employers must maintain confidential medical records on all employees for at least duration of employment plus 30 *years*. These records must include information about the employee's HBV vaccination status and a medical evaluation after any exposure incident.

Injury to Blood Vessels

This is fairly common, even for excellent acupuncturists. There are many points right next to blood vessels, such as in the popliteal crease at the back of the knee, Lung 9 at the wrist, Lung 5 at the cubital crease of the elbow. These are all right next to blood vessels. Deep needling, which we routinely do for sciatica type pain at the Gallbladder 30 point can puncture a blood vessel too. Sometimes it just happens.

You have 2 types of blood vessels – arteries and veins.
- Veins
  These are the easy ones. Apply direct pressure for 30 –

---

[4] As of 2019 in the US.

60 seconds with a dry, clean cotton ball to stop the bleeding.

You might be tempted to use alcohol. Don't. This thins the blood and promotes bleeding.

☯ Arteries
Less fun because they are so much higher in arterial pressure. The closer the needle site is to the heart, the higher the pressure will be.

If the needle is still in, remove it. Apply direct pressure with a clean, dry cotton ball for 5 minutes or until the bleeding stops. Sometimes you see a lump forming around the site under the skin – that's a bleed out from an arterial puncture. Apply pressure in the manner described above.

You also need to file an incident report.

Electrical Stimulation Safety

An electrical stimulation (e-stim) machine is similar to TENS units you might see in a chiropractor's office. It delivers a variable electrical current and can be great for relieving pain and moving stuck Qi and Blood and comes in a wide variety of styles to choose from. The leads from the unit attach to the handle of needles instead of to a pad like they do on a TENS unit, allowing us to deliver a mild electrical stimulation directly to affected tissues.

The use of e-stim does have some precautions, however.
☯ Do not use e-stim machines on patients with electrical implants like pacemakers.
☯ Do not use on heart patients
☯ Do not use on elderly patients

- Use with caution on patients with seizure disorders, as bioeclectical stimulation can disturb the brain and trigger a seizure.
- Do not span the heart
  Do not apply it to one side of the chest and to the other side of the chest across the heart. This can interfere with the normal internal electrical rhythm of the heart.
- Never crank the stimulation level up so high that it causes pain. Don't even come close. Adjust those levels in tiny tiny increments.
- Always use stainless steel needles with metal handles of a relatively thick gauge.
  Thinner needles can break with the pressure of e-stim on them.

Moxibustion Safety

You light this stuff on fire. Non-surprisingly, this can cause burns! Never, ever, ever leave moxa burning unattended. Don't leave the room. I mean it. Here are some other precautions, because you really need to avoid causing burns. Like really. This really pisses your patients off!

- Use extra precautions with patients who have neural injuries, diabetics, and anyone with pathologies resulting in paralysis.
- Indirect moxa precautions:
  This includes moxa sticks, moxa boxes, moxa on ginger or other substance, and any moxa application that doesn't come into direct contact with patient skin. Protect patient's skin from falling moxa and ashes.
- Direct moxa precautions
  Make sure patients have signed the written consent form that details the risks of direct moxa. Direct moxa is placed right on the patient's skin. Some practitioners like to do this for warming and fertility. Japanese style acupuncturists do this rather frequently too. Work with

your patient and ask them to tell you when it's feeling too hot. Remove quickly.

If your patient does sustain a burn from moxa, apply sterile gauze and a burn ointment. There are some awesome Chinese herbal burn ointments. I keep tubes of them in my office and use them for this. For a severe burn, consult a physician.

Bleeding Technique safety

You will learn plenty about this procedure in the future. For now, know that you need gloves, you need paper towels, hydrogen peroxide, and any of the blood spill kit stuff we mentioned before.

Some acupuncturists use 2 pair of gloves layered when they do bleeding.

Other acupuncture accidents you could encounter

This can include pain at or after the needle is inserted.

Pain

- ☯ Pain as the needles pierces the skin.
  This is often avoidable with careful and considerate insertion. Inserting too slowly *hurts*.
- ☯ Press the acupuncture guide tube to the skin and tap the top of the handle of the needle it in just firmly enough to get the top of the handle level with the top of the tube. This quickly gets the tip of the needle past the skin barrier before it even knows what's happening and avoids pain. And by the way, if you don't do this, the needle might fall over when you remove the tube and then you have to do it all over again.
- ☯ The closer you are to the ends of the extremities, the more nerve endings there are. Inserting on fingers, toes, hands, feet is always going to have a stronger sensation

than in the thigh or calf. One way to help is to massage the extremely local area where you are going to insert with your finger tip. That desensitizes the area so you can insert more easily and with less pain.

☯ It is always a bit painful when an artery is pierced. Or a nerve. When a patient has a sharp painful sensation or that fun electrical type of sensation, move that needle! You can lift the needle a little and reinsert at a different angle. Watch for blood causing a lump at the surface. If that happens, see the instructions above for blood vessel punctures.

☯ Pain at the needle site after insertion
Sometimes this happens because patients move around. Back the needle out a little, change the angle slightly and push it back to depth.

Needles can also get entwined in fibrous tissue. If that happens, rotate it back and forth gently until the fiber releases.

Patient Fainting
I've only had it happen a couple of times. Once was in a quit smoking clinic. I asked the woman if she was needle sensitive and she said no. I put 2 needles into one ear and she started to say she was dizzy, broke out in a cold sweat, and got very pale. Turns out she was indeed super needle sensitive.

☯ Usual signs and symptoms to watch for:
vertigo, dizziness, pallor, cold sweats, oppressive feeling in the chest, palpitation, nausea.
☯ Severe cases:
cold extremities, weak pulse, loss of consciousness, hypotension, and shock

How do you manage this situation?
- o Remove the needles immediately
- o Allow the patient to lie flat with the feet or legs slightly elevated to recover on his or her own.
- o Offer the patient warm drinks
- o Acupuncture treatment:
  Press or puncture GV26, PC6, LI4, ST36
- o Call for emergency medical assistance

This can be caused by nervous tension, hunger, fatigue, weakness in general, or overly forceful manipulation of the needle.

To prevent this situation in the first place, treat patients if they are tired, weak, fasting, or very nervous. Use gentle needle manipulation for these patients. And watch the patient closely. It's always better to catch them when they are *starting* to feel woozy than after they fall down!

Stuck Needles
Sometimes you inset a needle and find it is impossible to rotate it, lift and thrust it, or even withdraw it. This is generally caused by a muscle spasm or an aggressive needle manipulation. To manage this situation:
- o Relax the patient. Let them know you're going to take care of it.
- o Massage or tap the skin around the stuck needle.
- o Insert a point very close to this stuck needle. Inserting, tapping, and massaging spread out the Qi that is gripping the needle and allow you to remove it more easily.
- o If you know the needle is entangled in the fibrous tissue, try rotating it the other way.

Broken Needles

This is a sucky situation! Fortunately, it's rare. This is when the needle breaks off while it's in the skin. Usually, it breaks at the handle, which is why you never ever ever insert all the way to the handle!

This occurs more frequently with non-disposable needles after repeat use and sterilization. But it can also occur with poor quality needles, strong muscle spasms, excessive force in manipulation, or a change in the patient's position.

What do you do about it if it happens?
- Don't move the patient!
- If the broken part is still exposed, remove the needle with hemostats or forceps.
- If the needle broke subcutaneously, meaning nothing is sticking out, do *not* cut the skin! That's way way outside the scope of practice in the United States. Seek medical help immediately.

Injury to Lungs/Pneumothorax

I've had nightmares about this. When the lung tissue is punctured some of the alveoli collapse. This can cascade resulting in a collapse of part or all of the lung.

Needling on the chest, top of the shoulders, supraclavicular fossa, and upper back with perpendicular or nearly perpendicular deep needling can cause this.

Symptoms to watch for include the following. It should be noted that sometimes symptoms are delayed for several hours, even occurring once the patient gets home. If you see these in your clinic or if a patient calls you and says they have these s/sx, this could indicate a pneumothorax.

- Pain in the chest
- Cough
- **Dyspnea**
- **Pallor**
- **Cyanosis**
- **Coma**

If you see this *in* your clinic, remove the needles, encourage the patient to lie down calmly, and get them to a hospital. If you see the severe symptoms bolded above - dyspnea, pallor, cyanosis, coma - you *have* to call 911. And when the patient is safely in the ambulance, call your lawyer.

Injury to liver, spleen, or kidney

This can be caused by insertion that is too deep, with inappropriate manipulation, or wrong angle on the trunk of the body near the bottom and just below the bottom of the hypochondriac area on the front of the trunk, the lateral sides of the trunk and on the back.

Signs and symptoms of a liver or spleen puncture:
- Abdominal pain
- Rigidity of the abdominal muscles
- Rebound pain

Signs and symptoms of a kidney puncture:
- Pain in the lumbar region
- Tenderness and pain upon percussion
- Bloody urine
- Coma

These patients should immediately be taken to a hospital or you should call 911.

Injury to brain or spinal cord

This can be caused by insertion that is too deep or with inappropriate manipulation on points close to the brain or spinal cord. The back of the head, any area near a foramen in the skull, neck points, and nuchal ridges are all likely candidates for this. We often use these points for patients with stiff necks, for instance.

You will learn proper insertion techniques and angles for these points in your point location classes.

Signs and symptoms include convulsions, paralysis, and coma.

This is a 911 situation!
Take out the needles and call. Like, immediately.

I should also mention bent needles – it wasn't covered in my class, but I've had it happen a couple of times. Terrific fun. I was able to smoothly release the needle each time, but it took some doing. It can happen for a variety of reasons – patient shifting positions, falling asleep and jerking involuntarily, and strong muscle spasms.

And that, my friends, concludes the CNT and scare the bejesus out of you portion of our book!

Super Mega Bonus Material

You definitely need to work with your instructor and consult the most recent CNT manual for the most current procedures. Again, I cannot guarantee you that this scenario will get you a passing CNT exam.

It should be noted that the CNT exam doesn't really look like it does in clinic. You will probably have to show your ID and that you have a hard-sided kit. I used a cheap fishing tackle box from Academy. Small tool boxes work too. You will likely be expected to describe what is in the kit, but do not take it out and put it on the table. Everything stays in for now.

But all that said, this is what mine looked like.

1. Set up instruments and equipment.
2. It is important to say: I have washed my hands for 10 seconds, twice, with running water.
   (You say it verbally rather than doing it.)
3. When you set up the clean field towel, make sure it doesn't touch your clothes and that you pinch from dirty side, leaving clean side intact.
4. Put all of the Things you need onto the center of your clean field.

   Do not touch the stuff in the ziplock bags, but pour them out in a controlled manner, wiggling them out of the bag with your fingers while touching only the outside of the bag.

   Some instructors are less strict about this and say if you just washed your hands per CNT protocol, you should be able to remove stuff from your ziplock bags by reaching inside of it.

Prior to actually going to the CNT exam I was encouraged to separate the single-pack needles (they come 5 to a sheet), alcohol swabs, etc. Be sure to do your restock with clean hands. Clean your travel kit too. Everything should look squeaky clean when you take this exam.

Do not stack your items. If anything lands *outside* of the clean field, don't use it. If you goof, tell your examiner you goofed and what the proper procedure would be.

5. When you finish with the clean and sterile items, get out your sharps container and the waste bag. If right handed, put it on the right, if left handed put it on the left. Why? Because you don't want to cross over a clean field with contaminated stuff you're about to discard! As for the waste bag, don't put your hand *in* the bag to make stand up! Many examiners don't like you doing that.

    Don't include an antimicrobial hand cleaner for the test, and don't use the portable alcohol pumps either.

6. Next, clean your hands.
    Open 6-10 alcohol swabs and prep them for use. Don't do this over the clean field, but *off to the side* because you don't want to drip on the clean field.

    Tear 2 sides—making an L—open out so it sits up and swab doesn't wet the clean field. Put them near the bottom of the clean field. When you drop the waste into the waste bag, don't touch the edges of the bag!

7. This is the treatment part – you insert the needle. You will do this in a sitting position. Find a point on your

leg—the thigh recommended so you can see what you are doing.

Do all prep first. Roll up your pants leg, adjust hair, whatever. Then clean your hands with an alcohol swab—one swab per hand.

8. Clean the point to be needled. Be sure to let it dry. Don't contaminate the clean site after swabbing.

9. Instruction: Insert a 1" needle at least ¼ inch deep at 90 degree angle (if using a 1"needle, go in about 25% of needle shaft!), rotate needle clockwise 1 full turn.

    Drop the guide tube into the waste bag. Do the rotation (needle manipulation) using only the handle -don't touch the shaft with anything!

10. Remove needle, close insertion, dispose of used stuff.

    Withdraw the needle without touching the shaft or insertion site with your hands. Apply pressure to site with a clean cotton ball. Dispose of cotton, then "wash" hands with alcohol swab.

11. You are generally asked to repeat the steps from 7-10 again but with a 1.5 cun needle.

12. Packing it up.
    Properly repack unused clean/sterile equip. Properly dispose of all unused exposed needles (i.e., in your sharps container.) Properly dispose of all trash in your trash bag. Finally, properly return clean and contaminated containers to travel kit.

13. Tell the examiner you are going to wash your hands with water for 10 seconds, two times. . . sometimes the examiner prefers that you do an alcohol 'wash' instead.

They will let you know what the preferred procedures are in the pre-class that happens before the exam. Don't miss that pre-class!

Some final notes:

There are slight variations between examiners. When you sign up to take the CNT exam it's an all-day event. The first part of the day is a repeat of the CNT portions of this class. During the lecture part the person doing the lecture will demonstrate how to properly do a CNT procedure as above. This sets the standard for what you can do when you take the test yourself! Again:

Don't miss this portion of the CNT "Experience."

If you contaminate your clean field (like get it wet), before you do anything else, acknowledge your mistake to the examiner and tell them what should have happened. They will probably give you a chance to correct and do again. If so, repack whatever isn't contaminated and set up another clean field.
If you flat out fail one step, you don't need to continue. You'll have to do it again. You get 2 tries during the CNT exam, but you basically have to go to the back of the line in order to do it again.
Does all of this scare the hell out of you? It's actually lots less stressful than taking the test during the techniques class! The CNT exam wasn't so bad at all except I was nervous as all get out. Practice a lot. You'll be fine.

This page intentionally left blank.

SECTION 2
Needling Techniques

Now that you are familiar with clean needle technique and safety, you can get to the fun stuff!

This section is all about handling needles and interacting with Qi via the needle. Enjoy!

This page intentionally left blank.

Acupuncture Techniques 101 - Chapter 5

CHAPTER 6
Where This Came From
& Things to Know About Needles

Disclaimer: I am a serious history geek. I have a degree in it. Yeah. *That* geeky. I know history haters are rolling their eyes right now. But to me history is about the *story* part of the word. A crap ton of what I'm about to say will not be on any test you will ever take, but I think it's damned interesting stuff to know.

So. If you hate history, you can skip over this until you see the second big black header bar and we're cool. But it you like a good story, hang in there.

THE FREAKY COOL ANCIENT HISTORY OF OUR MEDICINE

Sometime between 200,000 years ago and 300,000 years ago our species was walking around the planet eating and getting eaten, talking, procreating, and fighting. Basically, the same things we do now, just without the iPhones.

About 65 million years before *that* happened a meteorite of fairly massive proportions smacked the crap out of the earth in what we now call the Shandong province in China. (Start in Los Angeles and drive west through the ocean until you reach Tokyo. Stop and have some sushi. Keep going through South Korea, go across the Yellow Sea just south of Beijing and you're there. Can't miss it.)

The mountain caused by this meteoric smack down contains big chunks of the rock that comprised it, which the ancient Chinese called "bian stone." At some point and for some reason, people began to mine this stuff and make musical instruments out of it.

It seemed that musicians who played these instruments lived a lot longer than those around them.

We now know that bian stone contains more than forty minerals and trace elements, can create FIR (far infra-red) waves, creates ultrasound type pulses in a range that is therapeutic for humans, and produces negative ions (think antioxidants – which slow the aging process).

What the ancient *Chinese* knew was that people who used this stone on a regular basis (like those musicians) were healthier and lived longer than their peers who did not. They also knew it could also be honed into super smooth edges, making it very effective for creating gua sha tools and needles. Bian stone (or "bian shi" in Chinese) needles have been found in Neolithic archeological excavations that date to about 6,000BCE, more than 8,000 years ago.

It seems kind of hilarious that crystal and stone healing is considered "new age" therapy, doesn't it? Not exactly new. But that's how it's gone in the course of our development. We learn cool stuff, forget about it, have to figure it out all over again, and then we call it "new."

And that's kind of what happened in China. The mountain from which this stone was mined was far from the Chinese court, difficult and dangerous to get to, and the stone itself was rare. Its use became scarce and it was nearly forgotten.

Nearly. The *Huangdi Nejing*, The Yellow Emperor's Classic, which details quite a lot about acupuncture was written between 475 and 221 BCE and speaks of these stones as well as nine different types of needles and multiple types of acupuncture therapies.

I should also mention that China might not be the only place that a theory resembling acupuncture and meridian systems developed. Ancient Ayurvedic writings from India detail a system of nadis which looks an awful lot like the meridian systems we study. And then there's the "ice man," Ötzi, who died around 5,300 years ago.[5] His body well preserved body was found along the border between Austria and Italy when the glacier there began to melt. His body was recovered in 1991 and has been studied heavily since then.

Ötzi has 61 tattoos, most of them now thought to be medical acupuncture markings to help treat his joint degeneration and chest pain, probably from the Lyme disease that researchers have found in his tissues.

What all of this comes down to is that this is a really, really old thing we are studying. And you're about to take your place in that ancient lineage. Welcome to history.

WHAT YOU NEED TO KNOW

Bian Stone. You need to know that. The first needles in use were made of stone, bone, and bamboo. The original use of needles was most likely to lance and drain boils, carbuncles, abscesses and the like. In eastern China where much of Chinese civilization developed, the climate was damp and hot, which increases the instances of these types of skin problems.

The *Huangdi Neijing*, written between 475 and 221 BCE, describes not only the use of bian stones, but also of nine different types of needles and the uses for each of them. These were filiform needles. Some were used for draining boils and abscesses, some to stimulate points on the skin, some for blood

---

[5] https://culturacolectiva.com/technology/otzi-the-iceman-tattoos-meaning

letting, etc. The *Neijing* also talks a lot methods for manipulating Qi via needle manipulation. And we're going to talk about some of that too.

TRADITIONAL TECHNIQUES

Metal needles obviously allow for greater flexibility in treatment and for a greater number of techniques. You will cover the *Neijing's* nine, twelve, and five needling methods in your advanced acupuncture technique classes. In this class we'll focus on how to insert, angles of insertion, stimulating the Qi, and tonifying and reducing techniques.

Nine needles from Neijing

Acupuncture doesn't add anything to the body, but stimulates points in order to open channels and stimulates organs in order to harmonize and regulate them. From a more modern perspective, it stimulates nerves, immune response, and helps relax the body.

The effects of treatment depend largely on the acupuncturists skills, ability to transmit Qi, and on the patient's reactions. Some patients are more sensitive to the external stimulation than others. Those who have high pain thresholds or are out of touch with their own bodies will have fewer noticeable sensations during treatment. Those who are sensitive will likely adjust and balance more quickly, but that's not a hard rule.

What we do during an acupuncture treatment is tonify deficiencies and reduce excesses to allow for better qi and blood flow through the meridians (see Chapter 10 for methods). Tonification points such as Stomach 36 can help push qi effectively in the body and even help the body build more qi.

Reducing techniques can help reduce the strength and amount of pathogens, phlegm, damp, etc.

MODERN TECHNIQUES

The beauty of acupuncture is that is adaptable and changeable, which I why it has been a viable form of medical treatment for 8,000+ years. Modern technology has made it's way into acupuncture in a variety of ways. Let's look at a few you are likely to use in clinic.

Modern Technique	Brief discussion
Electrical stimulation	Also called e-stim, this affects the bioelectric fields of the body. It is used for relaxation, stress reduction, releasing tight or overstrained muscles, and improving blood flow.
Magnetotherapy	This affects the electromagnetic fields of the body. Magnets are applied in the form of small beads under a small adhesive bandage at acupuncture point sites. It is often used on the ears, but can also be used in the form of bracelets and necklaces.
Heat lamps	That's what we usually call them in clinic, but they come in a couple of different varieties: • FIR (far infrared) lamps. These don't just warm, but help regulate body functions. They are inexpensive and are popular for home use. • TDP lamps. These go further than FIR lamps. They have an emission plate coated with multiple elements through which the heat is pushed. This mineral plate emits a different band of FIR energy which penetrates deeply. The cells of the body will absorb this more efficiently than near infrared.
Laser acupuncture	Popular with patients who cannot be needled. Also popular in veterinary acupuncture.
Sound wave acupuncture	This is the combination of sound and acupuncture and is still in its infancy, even though sound healing

	has long been a 'thing.' A system called Acutonics (there are others) uses a series of tuning forks instead of needles to stimulate the points and can have a strong effect. There are also special music tracks designed to target specific problems that are used in clinic.
Microsystem acupuncture	Microsystems are small compact areas of the body that reflect the *whole* body. Auricular acupuncture is one such system in which you can treat any part of the body by needling the ear.
Auricular acupuncture	Yes, already mentioned, but it's so popular and useful it gets its own spot on the table. It's frequently used in addiction treatment, but also for insomnia, pain, and stress reduction. Fun fact: right after I got my license I did a health fair targeting stress reduction via auricular acupuncture. I had 45 patients in a 2 hour period, most of whom didn't want stress reduction, but had everything else known to modern man wrong with them. All I had were ear needles, so that's all I did. I was amazed at how much better everyone felt afterwards, despite not deploying a single TCM point the whole evening! Powerful stuff.
Scalp acupuncture	There are a couple of systems of scalp acupuncture. They are often used in neurological disease to affect brain function. There are also "motor" lines on the side of the head to help with movement issues in the extremities and head, assist with balance and hearing issues and more. These are also used frequently in post-stroke treatment.
Hand acupuncture	There are a couple of different types of hand acupuncture systems too. The Koryo hand system is probably the most well known. This is another form of microsystem acupuncture.

And there is so much more waiting for you!

OK. Now that we've talked about the history of acupuncture, traditional and modern techniques, let's get into the needle itself.

Tail   Handle   Root   Body/shaft   Tip

Part	Brief discussion
Tail	Far end of the handle. Many needles don't have this 'decoration.' Doesn't matter much, though can help hold moxa.
Handle	Texture and grip is often dependent upon personal taste. The needle shown above is a spring handle – named for the coiled shape. These types are good for general acupuncture, e-stim, moxa/warm needle. Some needles have a spiraled handle like this, some are smooth, and a very popular Japanese type called a Seirin has a plastic handle.
Root	End of the handle, closest to the shaft.
Body or shaft	Part of this will be inserted into the skin. Not the whole thing – never insert all the way to the root.
Tip	This is the part that comes into contact with the skin first. It should be very sharp and thin – mosquito-like, in that you don't feel it much when it pierces the skin.

Needle length and gauges

Needles come in different lengths and thickness (gauges). The length/gauge combination you choose depends largely on where you are needling.

Gauges can be a little confusing to the math challenged such as myself. In the Chinese system of needle measurements, the bigger the number, the thinner the needle. If you are buying Japanese needles, it's just the opposite.

Choose your gauge based on the type of stimulation you want to do and how sensitive your patient is. While some patient populations seem to be very "no pain, no gain," in their approach to getting treatment, US patients are generally pain averse, so they prefer thinner gauge needles and very smooth needles (like Seirins).

As a rule, he thicker the needle, the more likely the patient is to feel the sensations more acutely.

You will usually see the gauge first on a box of needles, then the mm or cun designation.

Needle length guides

Cun measure		Millimeter measure
0.5 cun	=	15mm
1.0 cun	=	25 or 30mm*
1.5 cun	=	40mm
2.0 cun	=	50mm
2.5 cun	=	65mm
3.0 cun	=	75mm
4.0 cun	=	100mm

*Both of these are considered to be 1 cun needles.

Gauge/thickness guides

Read these across for equivalency. No. 32 in the Chinese system, for instance, is 0.25 to 0.26 in diameter and is the same as the Japanese No. 5 needle.

Chinese No.	Diameter (cm)	Japanese No.
28	0.38	--
30	0.32/0.30	8
32	0.25/0.26	5
34	0.22	
36	0.20	3
38	0.18	2
40	0.16	1
42	0.14	01
44	0.12	02

As a general rule:
- ☯ 0.5 cun needles (15mm) are used for the ear, face, and sometimes fingers/toes.
- ☯ 1 cun needles are the more common, workhorse, everyday kind of needle. These are what you will likely use in most treatments.
- ☯ 1.5 cun (40mm) length needles are also commonly seen in clinics. It's a personal preference and depth of treatment thing.
- ☯ Needles in the 3-5 cun range are used for big muscular areas like the gluteal tissues (great for treating sciatica) and for a technique called threading
- ☯ Use 42 and 44 gauge needles (01 and 02 in the Japanese system) for needle sensitive patients and in areas with great sensitivity – like fingers, toes, hands, feet, wrist and ankle, lip area, etc. Anywhere there are many, tightly packed sensory nerve endings, basically.

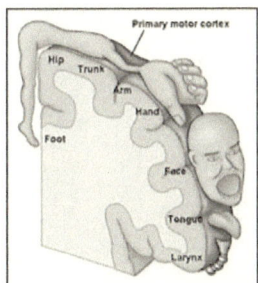

Have you seen this homunculus illustration? This is designed to teach you where the sensory input goes, but I use it as a general guide as to the sensitivity of an area when I teach. The bigger the body part in this strange looking illustration, the more nerve endings are packed into that area. The more nerve endings, the more likely the patient is to experience pain if you needle there.

I do find that the feet are more sensitive than indicated, though less so than the hand.

This page intentionally left blank.

CHAPTER 7
Preparing to Needle

You're probably thinking, "let's get on with this already!" And I hear you. By now you've likely bought all the fun toys and goodies you need for your portable acupuncture kit. My first week I was given a shopping list, I went into our student store and herbal dispensary, bought needles in various sizes and pack combinsations, moxibustion materials, cups, a gua sha tool or two, some oil, and other goodies.

I was absolutely itching to start poking holes in something living (not my cats – they know where I sleep), but Dr. Qiu was insistent that we first learn to prepare ourselves and to practice on oranges (I thought those were the closest to the feel of needling living tissues), needling practice cushions, several layers of paper towels, etc. I recommend you do likewise for a while.

Your instructor should show you how to do this and help you learn to practice on inanimate objects before needling a human being.

PREPARING YOURSELF TO NEEDLE

In addition to practicing on non-living things, you need to build strong hands with good muscle memory to treat with acupuncture. Hence all that practice holding and inserting a needle. But you also need *strong Qi*.

If you have not studied qigong, you may not know this, but there are three regulations you do to govern and strengthen your own Qi flow. These regulations will also calm you down a helluvalot before tests!

These are regulation of the body, breath and mind.

Body	Calm your body, relax your muscles, let your spine be upright (not board straight – you need those natural curves!) so that your cerebro spinal fluid flows easily. This also allows you to breathe more easily and makes it possible for your Qi to flow smoothly. You can do this sitting or standing, but I recommend standing with feet about hip-width apart.
Breath	Let your breath slow as your body relaxes. Let your breathing slow a little, and let it get a little deeper. Breathe in to a count of four, hold for a count of four, exhale to a count of four. That can be as slow or fast as you need it to be. Don't make yourself feel breathless!
Mind	Relax your mind. Drop your worries, anxieties, anger, and anything doesn't serve you. Tune in to your breathing and the relaxation in you body.

Do one of these at a time, in this order. You breath is the key here. It will help calm your mind. Shallow breathing triggers anxieties and triggers the sympathetic (fight/flight/freeze) system; deeper, more relaxed, slower breathing helps relax your body and mind and lets you drop into your parasympathetic nervous system.

Strengthening your finger force for needling

First, do the three regulations above. Do them for between 3 and 10 minutes and noticed what feels different.

Next, do this exercise.
1. While in your lovely regulated Qigong state, visualize lines of light moving up from the earth below you and into your legs, all the way into your abdomen. Let this flow as slow or fast as feels correct to your body.

If you don't *feel* anything, imagine it. Let yourself play make-believe like you might have as a child. Your Qi will follow your thought, so pretend away because that will actually make it happen.

2. Let that light come up into our chest and surround your heart. Imagine it making a larger and larger sphere around your heart and lungs, expanding in front and to the sides and to the back as well.

3. Let your hands "float" upward in a relaxed way from the sides of your body with your *palms down*. Bend your elbows so that both of your hands come toward your heart with the palms still down.
4. On the next slow, deep inhale, keeping your palms flat, down, and parallel to the ground, but reach outward toward the horizon so that your arms are out to either side of your body.

    Visualize the light that is filling your chest spreading out to your downward facing palms.

5. Hold for a moment, then exhale, bringing your hands back to the spot in front of Ren 17 (in front of your heart). As you do so, imagine/visualize the light coming back from your hands and into your shoulders and chest.

Repeat this a number of times. No set amount, but if you need an amount, I recommend 36 cycles. It adds up to nine and is a good number in Chinese philosophy. It was a stock answer from most Qigong teachers, though Master Junfeng Li said "do until it feels good in your body, in your mind."

If you do this before each needling session, your treatments will strengthen immensely, your needle force will be great, you'll connect with the patient's Qi more readily and effectively. And your car payments will magically lower. OK, I made that last one up. But the rest is true.

I used to do this in the mornings before my first patient, treat all morning, go to lunch and do it again before the afternoon patients. So it's not like you have to do this before *every* patient.

Practice palpating for points

When you learn point locations you get pretty detailed instructions about where the points are. You need to memorize the stuffing out of that because you're going to need it for any exam you take in point locations, for a whole bunch of the energetics tests, and for a bunch of board questions.

BUT those are just guidelines as to where the points are. People aren't machines or robots. They are individuals with unique biology and exactly where you find *their* points may be slightly different than what your books say.

For this reason you need to treat thoughtfully and part of that is palpating around the book location gently to find the location of the actual point on that human body. This takes a lot of practice.

This is part of the reason I do the three regulations before my first patients of the morning and afternoon. I can *feel* the Qi of the point when I palpate lightly and that's where I needle even if it isn't exactly where Peter Deadman's book says the point is.

I will say, the point is always very close to the described location, so if you find you're even as little as a cun off the mark, then you're probably on a different point entirely.

Open your favorite point location book up and look at Heart 4, 5, 6 and 7 for example. Those are extremely close together as are the Ren points and Kidney points on the abdomen and lower abdomen. Can't stray too far off the path!

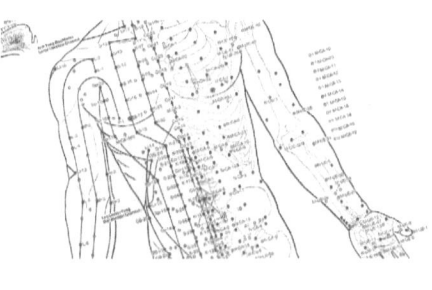

Do this often and eventually you will either just find your fingers are drawn to the correct point or you might actually see it. It's like building a muscle memory in a way, but it's also a Qi type memory.

Now you're prepared to needle. If you've done all this, your Shen is regulated. You're good to go.

Bonus pre-treatment Qigong routine that absolutely no one is going to test you on

If you enjoyed the Qigong exercise, try this one. I like it for pre-treatment and just for life in general. It's a lovely way to start a day.

- ☯ Stand with your feet apart and relax your body visualizing your cells opening up and away from each other a little so your own Qi flows more easily.

- ☯ Begin to inhale and lift your arms out from your sides palms up and visualize (or pretend or whatever words work for you) gathering Qi from both near to you and *very* far away. See it sticking to your hands as you continue to lift your hands up, arms out and elbows softly bent – not rigid.

- ☯ When your arms arc up so they are parallel to each other, palms facing each other and straight over your shoulders gently face your palms down, level with the floor, fingertips pointing toward each other. Begin to exhale and bring your palms down the plane of your body – basically down your Stomach meridian.

  As you exhale and lower your hands down the Stomach meridian, visualize/imagie Qi entering the top of your head and flowing down your body into the lower Dantian, which is the core of your body about 2 inches below your belly button and in the center of your body from front to back.

- ☯ Bring your flat palms all the way down to your lower abdomen so that your elbows are gently bent and facing out. You should be finishing your exhale at this point.

☯ Turn your palms out and move your arms out repeat this cycle.

☯ Do this 3-6 times. Move at a comfortably slowly speed – comfortable for you might look different than for someone else in your cohort. There is no right or wrong.

This page intentionally left blank.
Actually, it's full of Qi, you just can't see it yet. ☺

CHAPTER 8
Wielding the Needle

This chapter covers holding the needle, proper angles of insertion and needle direction that will keep your patient safe, two hand and one hand needling technique, depth of insertion, and withdrawing the needle.

HOLDING THE NEEDLE

Hold the needle in whatever your dominant hand is. If you are left handed, hold the needle in your left hand. If you are right handed....well, you probably get what I'm talking about.

I've heard that holding a needle is like holding the tail of a tiger. You have to hold it tightly enough so it doesn't move, but always remember to watch the tiger. The tail in this analogy is the needle. The tiger is the patient.

While holding the needle/guide tube in your dominant hand, find the point (and of course you are using CNT), and steady the needle. Be one with the needle, grasshopper. See it as an extension of your own Qi. Watch the patient (the tiger). Use both hands whenever possible. This gives more flexibility and control, especially when you tap the needle in.

Sometimes, however you have to use the "pressing" hand (your non-dominant hand) to guide the Qi to the point, to tap on the point or along channel or to fix a blood vessel/tendon in place.

Actually, your whole body's posture should be comfortable and balanced. Qi should flow from your Dantian to your arm, then to point. Get your whole body involved. If you have no feeling of Qi, adjust your posture, move closer, etc.

Let's peel that apart a little more and look at holding the needle.

Two hand and one hand techniques

Two hand technique

This is how you will insert most of the time.

Hold the guide tube with your non-dominant hand, tap the needle in firmly but not hard with your dominant hand.

Remove the guide tube and hold the handle of the needle with your thumb, index and middle fingers and maybe your ring finger too. This depends upon your comfort, your Qi, your hand strength, your finger size and more.

Using the best grip for you, you will then insert the needle a little deeper and/or manipulate the needle. You will also use the same finger grip to remove the needles at the end of the session.

One handed technique

Some points require you to hold the guide tube and tap the needle in with one hand. LU 7 for instance, requires that you pinch the area while you are inserting the needle.

To do a one-hand insert, hold the top of guide tube with your middle, ring finger and thumb then use your index finger to tap it in.

Remove the guide tube with the same hand and hold it in your palm with your little and ring fingers. Use your index, middle finger, and thumb to complete the insert and/or manipulate the needle just as you do in the two-hand insertion.

There are a couple of one-handed techniques to talk about.

One-handed technique	What that looks like
Pressing	Inserting the needle with your dominant hand while using the index finger of your non-dominant hand to press at the site of the insertion point.

Why would you want to do this? Some points are very close to arteries, blood vessels, tendons or nerves. You want to be sure you don't hit one of these features, so you use the index finger of your non-dominant hand to locate it, the press it just hard enough to keep it out of the way. Hold your finger there while you insert the needle and push it into place. You don't want to pull the skin while you are doing this.

Some examples:
- LU 9. This point is between the radial artery and the bone. Press on the artery to keep from needling it, insert the needle to depth, then remove your pressing finger.
- P6 has a tendon very near it. Fix the tendon in place with your pressing index finger, insert the needle and push it to the proper depth. Now remove your pressing finger. |
| Holding | Using the dominant hand to control the insertion while using the non-dominant hand to hold the shaft of the needle.

Use your non-dominant hand to hold the needle guide tube while the dominant hand controls tapping the needle into the skin. Remove the guide tube with the non-dominant hand and hold the handle of the needle with the dominant hand. Put the guide tube down and pick up a |

One-handed technique	What that looks like
	square of clean gauze. Wrap the clean side which you have not touched around the shaft of the needle. Now using both hands in synchronized parallel movement, press down to insert the needle. You may need to move the guaze further up the shaft then press down with both hands again until the needle has reached depth. Why would you want to do this? This technique is used for very long needles which tend to bow when you attempt to insert them with just one hand. GB 30 is an example: this is a point used to treat sciatic pain and generally takes a 2-3 cun needle.
Stretching	Stretching the skin with the fingers of the non-dominant hand (usually the thumb and index finger) while using the dominant hand to insert the needle using the one-handed technique. Continue to stretch until the needle is inserted to proper depth. Why would you want to do this? It is really useful for wrinkly areas (older people), areas of loose skin (such as after child birth), on the abdomen or whereever there is a lot of give to the skin and not much muscle structure to support it underneath.
Pinching	Pinching is a technique in which you use the non-dominant hand to pinch the skin up (again, thumb and index finger) and then use the dominant hand to insert the needle using the one-handed technique. Keep pinching the skin until the needle is inserted to proper depth. Why would you want to do this? This technique is very useful wherever the skin and muscle is very thin over the bone. This way

One-handed technique	What that looks like
	the skin isn't too tight to impede the insertion and the needle doesn't hit the bone when you insert (which hurts wicked bad). I've seen it used most often at Yintang (a popular extra point which is right between the eyebrows), Yuyao (an extra point in the middle of the eyebrow), and Lung 7. It isn't often used on the scalp because there's not much to pinch there (scalp acupuncture uses a transverse insertion you will learn in Advanced Acupuncture Techniques I.)

ANGLES OF INSERTION

The angle of insertion is very important for both the acupuncture point you are using and for the underlying musculature, vessel, bone, and organ structure. Always learn the proper angles of insertion so that you will do no harm to your patients.

When an angle of insertion is given in acupuncture classes or in acupuncture books, these angles are relative to the plane of the skin of the patient. "Perpendicular" for 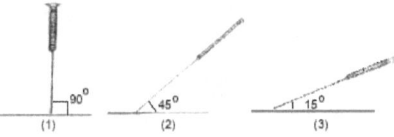 instance is perpendicular to the patient's skin at the point of insertion rather than perpendicular to the treatment table or the plane of the earth.

Insertion Angle	Areas appropriate for this angle
Transverse or horizontal angle 15 - 25°	• In very thin areas or where there isn't much muscle. Scalp acupuncture would be an example of a very thin area. Scalp acupuncture has several "lines" that are longer than any needles you can use. Rather than using one long needle, several are inserted transversely along the line. Lung 7 is another place you use transverse needling (along with the pinching technique covered above) as it is over the bone and there is not enough tissue to insert any other way. • Over organs Over the Lung area (both anterior and posterior surfaces) for instance. • Next to the mouth You don't want to needle into the mouth cavity, so insert transversely. Some nasty bacteria can live in the mouth cavity. You don't want that transferring into the skin of the surrounding tissues. • Between the fingers, along the spaces between two bones.
Oblique angle 45°	Oblique insertion is appropriate in thinner areas such as the chest, abdomen, intercostal muscle spaces, into the back muscles in the thoracic areas or anywhere there is a danger of hitting an organ or nerve. This is especially important in thinner patients. Please note that as you descend down the back you can insert more perpendicularly until you get down to the L2 area when you can insert fully perpendicularly.
Perpendicular angle 90°	This is the general purpose angle that, unless otherwise specified, is used for *most* points. On the lower back in the lumbar area from about L2 and downward you can safely insert at a perpendicular

Insertion Angle	Areas appropriate for this angle
	angle due to the thickness of the musculature in this area.

DIRECTIONS OF INSERTION

There are two ways to think of this: 1) You needle as the point is related to the human anatomy around and underlying it, 2) You needle the point as it is related to the disease you are treating.

In regard to needling relating to the disease treated, you angle the needle toward the affected area. You guide the needle and thus the Qi to areas you would like to affect. (Example: treating urinary incontinence—angle needle downward toward this area.)

But even when you are doing that, you must keep in mind the underlying anatomical structure. Here is what I'm talking about.

Anatomy	Direction of Insertion
Head	In general: horizontal – perpendicular to the skin. You can direct anteriorly, posteriorly, laterally or at an angle in relation to the point of insertion. Often you are directing the Qi *toward* the site of a disease or *away* from the site of a disease and this will determine the direction of the insertion on the head. The Yuyao point, an extra point on the eyebrow, for instance can be used for eyelid twitching so you might want to aim it at the twitch. You might have a patient with nasal congestion or sinus problems so you might aim LI 20 or Bitong toward the nose. If you aren't directing the Qi specifically, do what is easiest. For instance, if you are needling Du 20 and aren't directing the Qi somewhere and you patient is supine (face up on the table), angle the needle toward the back of the head. If the patient is prone (face down), angle the needle toward the front of the head.

Anatomy	Direction of Insertion
Face	In general: horizontal to the skin after insertion. Needles on the face can also be directed toward a manifestation (congestion, twitch, palsy, etc.) and so may be directed anteriorly, posteriorly, or at some angle. You'll see this commonly with Yintang which is often directed downward, with Bitong which is often directed toward the nose, etc.
Chest along midline	In general: horizontal to the surface of the skin and downward. Often directed downward on the sternum. This is a shallow area, so you insert obliquely or transverse-oblique here, but this is also a strong point affecting the Lung and Qi. Since you want Lung Qi to descend, you angle the needle downward.
Chest lateral to the midline	In other words – anywhere not protected by the sternum. In general: oblique or horizontal angle and outward toward the lateral sides of the body Needles in this area should be angled toward the outward edge of the body, following the body curve so that you are not angling the needle toward the Lung or other organ.
Upper and middle back	In general: oblique insertion. The direction the needles are angled depends upon the location of insertion. Needles on the first Bladder line, 1.5 cun from the posterior midline for instance are angled inward medially. Needles on the second Bladder line, 3 cun from the posterior midline are angled laterally. Needles inserted on the Du channel, the posterior midline, are angled depending upon the angles of the spinous processes of the vertebrae.

Anatomy	Direction of Insertion
Abdomen	Often inserted perpendicularly, but not deeply.
Lower back	Mostly inserted perpendicularly in the lumbar spine region and on the gluteal muscles.
Four limbs	Inserted perpendicularly except in thin areas (Lung 7, for instance or Kidney 6).

DEPTH OF INSERTION

How deep you insert a needle depends on several factors and is relative to these factors.

Factor	Discussion
Age	• Children are small. Shallower insertion. • Old people shrink, shrivel, spaces between discs shrink. Shallower insertion.
Constitution	• Big person (either fat big or muscle big or constitutionally big) versus little person (thin, small constitution, lean) for example. Bigger people can take deeper insertion. • Smaller people need a shallower insertion. Insertion depth is relative to constitution, muscle development, overall size, etc.
Area	• Take into consideration the part of the body you are needling and what lies underneath. Also factor in how much muscle is here, and the depth you have to go to get Qi sensation.
Disease condition	• For skin problems: shallow • For bone problem: needle close to bone • Steaming bones sensation: deeply • Blood deficiencies or chronic problems: deeper than not • External problems: shallower
Season and weather condition	• In the Spring and Summer the Qi wants to go surface because Yang is up. The Qi will be more superficial at these times. Needle shallowly.

Factor	Discussion
	• In the Winter and Fall the Qi hides inside the body more because Yin is strongest and Yin is deep in quality. Needle more deeply to connect with the Qi. • Sunny or rainy days also make a difference. When the weather is sunny, the Qi is up because these days are more Yang so you can needle more shallowly. On rainy or cool days the Qi is more inward because these days are more Yin, so needle more deeply.
Patient sensitivity	• Some patients are more needle-sensitive than others so they will get a Qi sensation more shallowly. Others are less sensitive so you may have to go deeper and maybe even manipulate more in order for them to get the sensation.

WITHDRAWL OF NEEDLES

Though some practitioners will hire acupuncture assistants to do this, I consider it part of the treatment, so I like to do this myself. I feel it gives the patient a sense of closure too.

After you have retained the needles for the recommended time, regulate your Shen – quiet your mind, regulate your body, breath, and mind. When you place your hand on the needle to withdraw it, pay attention to whether needle is grabbed by muscle. I recommend you see the needle as an extension of yourself again and feel down into the needle for how it has interacted with the tissue below.

If it feels a little "stuck" do this:
- ☯ Manipulate the needle until sensation is loose
- ☯ Lift needle to the subcutaneous level
- ☯ Withdraw the needle.

Close the hole or no?
You have 2 choices here: close the hole or leave it open.

Closing the hole means energetically closing the tiny wound you made in the skin. Most of the time that's what you want to do so the patient's Qi doesn't leak or leave them open to energetic interference. Frankly, from a purely physical standpoint, it also gives you a chance to quickly inspect the skin for bleeding or subcutaneous leakage and count your needles as you remove. It's also a nice thing to do and completes the treatment.

But sometimes you want to leave the hole open. There is a part of the Neijing that talks about "wagging the tail" upon insertion to release toxic heat. If that is what you are treating, you want to do that to give the heat a way out of the body.

But usually you close the hole. Here's how.

To close the hole withdraw the needle and then press the site of insertion with a clean, dry cotton ball. I give it a little clockwise twist like I'm pushing a round cover over the hole.

If there is a little bleeding, press with the cotton ball until it stops then toss the cotton ball per CNT regulations.

Do we really fill up our hazardous waste containers with cotton balls? No, not really. By federal standards, you only have to do that if you could squeeze the cotton ball and fluid dripped out. We usually put it into the waste bin.

If the cotton ball is still clean and there is no bleeding or fluid, you can use it again for the next closing/withdrawl.

If you want to leave the hole open you would shake the needle gently to symbolically enlarge the hole so toxins or heat can release. Don't do that for now. You'll get there when you study the *Neijing* methods in the advanced acupuncture techniques course.

ORDER OF INSERTION AND REMOVAL

In general, most of us insert from the top of the body downward and from the middle outward, though there are different orders of insertion you will learn later for specific techniques.

In general:

- ☯ Insert these first. Obviously you won't use all of these in each treatment, but if they show up in your treatment pattern, they get priority in this order:
    - o Du 20, Ren 17, Ren 6
    - o Lung 1, Stomach 17, Liver 14, Large Intestine 11, Lung 7
    - o Do any side points or limb points after these.

- ☯ Removal is in the same basic order.

In reality? Yeah, I often do these point in this order unless I know I have some points that are going to be sensitive or painful. Kidney 1 for instance, on the bottom of the foot. Inserting this point without pain takes some finesse - more on that in your point location texts. I've got a good method - better than most I think, and I almost see people smile and hear them say, "Man, that was a *lot* less painful than I was afraid it would be!"

I digress. If you have points you know are going to be less than pleasant, get them out of the way first if you can. Patients remember what you did *last* in the treatment, not first. So do the happy stuff last – like give them a quick reflexology treatment or some relaxing tuina. My favorite clinic supervisor, Dr.

Xiaotian Shen,[6] taught me this trick. He did 10 minutes of tuina for almost every patient and while he was doing it he would smoothly say, "Can I book you for a treatment at this same time next week or would another time be more convenient for you?" They almost always rebooked for the following week. He had an app on his phone tied to his clinic booking system so he'd rebook them before he left the room and say, "I set up next week's appointment for you. See you next week! You can up and get dressed when you're ready. You're all done!"

He also collected payment up front so there was basically nothing else for the patient to do except say goodbye to the receptionist and float off to their vehicles in a happy cloud.

Dr. Shen is brilliant, I tell you.

---

[6] https://aoma.edu/about/faculty/xiaotian-shen-md-mph-lac

This page intentionally left blank.
Draw me a picture or something.

Acupuncture Techniques 101 - Chapter 8

CHAPTER 9
Needle Manipulation

The point of acupuncture (sorry, bad pun) is not just to poke holes in people, but to use the needles to bring Qi to the area so that the patient gets benefits from the tratment. This brings therapeutic effect and is the foundation of the tonifying and reducing methods (see Chapter 10 for more information). The basic principles of tonification and reducing (also called sedation in TCM) are:

- ☯ If there are deficiencies, tonify
- ☯ If there is excess, fullness or stagnant, use a reducing technique

Using any technique without the patient getting Qi sensation at the site of the acupuncture needles is rather pointless (again sorry, bad pun).

When you insert a needle and it reaches the level in the body where there is Qi, then you get the Qi sensation. When you first tap needle into the dermis you might feel a little something but it's probably not qi.

You need to go to the level of Qi to feel the Qi sensation. The Peter Deadman[7] and CAM[8] books define where the various level of Qi will be for the points. Bear in mind that levels of Qi can vary from patient to patient, from season to season and according to weather as discussed in the previous class.

---

[7] Deadman, A Manual of Acupuncture, 2nd ed., ISBN 0951054651
[8] Cheng, Chinese Acupuncture and Moxibustion, 3rd ed., ISBN 7119059947

That said, you may encounter schools of thought that deviate from this manner of thinking. Some say that the physical body is just one level of the total energetic body and as such any insertion, as long as the needle will stand on it's own, is reaching some level of Qi and is thus beneficial for the patient. Some Japanese acupuncture techniques use a stylus rather than a needle to touch the points instead of inserting a needle, stating that stimulation without insertion is a better technique. Even within TCM there are points which are said to work better with acupressure – no insertion at all – than with acupuncture.

We're here to learn the TCM stuff, obviously, so yes, memorize the standard stuff taught here, but remember that other cultures and philosophies of acupuncture will promote different methods from what we learn.

ARRIVAL OF QI

Now that the needle is in, you're looking for Qi to come and meet that needle you inserted. This is what gives the therapeutic effect in acupuncture and is the foundation of the tonifying and reducing methods we talk about in Chapter 10.

How do you know when the Qi has arrived? Two ways: the sensations the patient feels and the sensations you as the practitioner feel.

Patient Sensations

These vary from patient to patient, but many report these common feelings at the needling site when the Qi arrives:
- Sore sensation
- Aching
- Numbness
- Heaviness
- Distention
- Radiating sensation like water flowing or energy opening

Sensations could be slow or fast, gentle, radiating. There might be no sensation at the local area, but sensation at the distal area from point. I've had a patient recently who said they felt something heavy on the medial side of their big toenail when I inserted a needle at Liver 3. That makes sense, as this is where the Liver channel originates. Patients might say they feel the channel "light up" or feel a surge of energy down the channel. Sometimes they indicate that there is a warm sensation.

In regard to pain, some points might indeed hurt, especially at the ends of fingers and toes. The aforementioned Liver 3 can be an unpleasant sensation too. Pain is often felt right at insertion, but goes away rapidly. I ask people if the needle has settled in or quit hurting and the answer is usually yes.

If it doesn't but isn't really painful, you can often tap around the point or tap up the channel either with one finger or in a "drumming" pattern with several fingers. Visualize smoothing out blockages in the channel and this can make the sensation smooth out for them.

Sensitive patients might need a shallow insertion—some people can even get acupressure benefits equal to acupuncture benefits.

A good qi sensation might ache, but it will do so somewhat comfortably, like a good stretch on a tight muscle. Sensation of Qi might be hard to explain if patient has never felt Qi, done qigong, etc. but they usually get the hang of it quickly.

There are styles of acupuncture that don't require that the patient get sensation. As mentioned previously, some Japanese styles only require the practitioner to feel sensation. Needling styles in this mode of treatment are very shallow and cause nothing unpleasant for the patient. This is a qigong-like acupuncture type treatment, though it uses different terminologies than qigong. Those practitioners need to concentrate on sensation of their own bodies and need to strongly extend their own qi into the needles.

Not Qi, not good sensations

- Nerve sensations
  If your patient feels an electrical type sensation that hurts or buzzes, this can be the needle touching or coming far too close to a nerve. This is *not* Qi sensation, but you touching their nerves! This feels like the sensation of hitting your elbow on the "funny bone" and getting that uncomfortable jolt sensation. I've seen this happen with deep needling at the GB 31 point on the gluteus muscles when treating sciatica, for instance. When the patient feels this electrical sensation, back that needle up a little or redirect it. Don't manipulate too much around these areas!

- Blood vessels
  This is painful and is often a sharp pain that makes the patient jump. Stop! Do not needle through that!

  You as the needler might feel resistance when you touch a blood vessel. If you push through it you will feel an emptiness then you'll start to notice surface or subcutaneous bleeding. Stop! Remove the needle and press with a cotton ball until bleeding stops.

- Muscle
  OK, not really so bad. Lots of acupuncture points are located within muscle tissue. This might feel heavy to the patient or distended. There are nerve endings within the muscles, so watch for numbness, that electrical sensation, etc.

- Bone

  If you hit bone, this hurts and feels like a deep ache. It can be sharp as well, depending on the nerve concentration at the surface of the bone. Some systems of acupuncture actually require that you barely touch the bone and then back the needle off, so this isn't necessarily a crime. But if you insert too quickly, too hard, too deeply this can really hurt and that's not good.

Practitioner Sensations

What about how *you* feel the arrival of Qi at the insertion point? Most commonly you, the practitioner, feel a tightness or vibration. Where there is muscle, you may feel the muscle grab the needle giving a resistance, tightness, or "biting the bait" feeling. If you don't feel a strong grab, you might feel a vibration.

What if you feel nothing?
- First, cut yourself some slack. You're new here.
- Do Qigong exercises before you do this.
- Concentrate just on the needle and notice what you feel. Don't push it. Just continue to really focus in on the needle in your fingers and what you feel coming back through it.
- Practice a lot. Insert at known acupuncture points – Stomach 36 is a good candidate. Lots of Qi here and most of us need a good Spleen and Stomach tonification!

Very sensitive practitioners can feel sensation at the organ or area at which treatment is aimed. They might feel the Qi with fingers, in the body, or intuitively. I've known a few who could see it. How you sense it will depend on you.

There are some factors on both the practitioner's part and on the patient's part that can slow or negate the arrival of Qi.

Practitioner Factors	Discussion
Poor point location	Qi travels through the meridians along set pathways to set points. If your point location is inaccurate, you can manipulate the needle all you want and nothing will happen.
Improper depth	If the needle tip stops too shallow or too deep, you will miss the level at which Qi flows at this point. If you go too deep the patient might feel Qi for a moment and then lose the sensation. If you are too shallow, then nothing happens. The more common error here for newbies is the latter – too shallow.
Imperfect manipulation	You're simply not doing it right somehow. More on specific techniques in a moment.
Imperfect treatment environment	Too hot, too cold, too uncomfortable, too much noise – things that the patient just can't get past to relax. This depends a lot on the patient and the culture they come from. In many parts of the world where culture is very communal people can relax in the midst of a sea of their peers who are all talking, laughing, and getting acupuncture. In the US it's more common to have a quiet environment, individual experiences, soft music, etc. even in community clinic settings.
Patient Factors	Discussion
Weak constitution	Sometimes, no matter how good you are, can't make it happen. Constitution may be too weak— can use other methods to tonify rather than acupuncture. Herbs and nutrition are the keys to strengthen patient constitution.
Needle insensitive	People with high pain thresholds, for instance. Sometimes this is because they are disconnected

	from their bodies; sometimes this is genetic. Red headed patients (natural ones, not bottle red-heads), for instance, often have a very high tolerance for pain and a resistance to pharmaceutical sedation. They can also be very needle insensitive.

METHODS FOR PROMOTING QI

There are a few things you can do to correct it most of the time. Try these methods of you are having trouble getting the Qi at the needle site.

- Adjust location and depth.
  You can also adjust needle angle as long as this sensation is not too strong. You don't want your patient tensing up against the sensation.

- Wait for the Qi.
  Sometimes Qi is slow to arrive. Check your point location and depth – if it seems fine, wait a bit.

- Tonifying Qi or weak patients
  As discussed above, constitutionally weak patients may not have enough strength for the Qi to arrive well or for them to feel it if it does. You can tonify using other methods – diet, herbs, Qigong.

- Manipulate the needle
  There are specific needle manipulations you can do to help the Qi arrive. You can adjust the intensity of the manipulation, usually making it stronger. You can also direct the Qi sensation toward the affected organ or area and might feel a difference that way.

METHODS OF MANIPULATION

The talk of manipulation begs the question of how you do that. First, it's very important to first regulate your own Qi. Once you have done that, you must then make the needle an extension of your hand.

Move the Qi from your lower Dantian to your whole body, specifically to your hand. Move your Qi down the needle. Feel the tip as you manipulate it. This is covered in Chapter 7. You'd do yourself and your patients a tremendous favor if you take Qigong classes. This helps you forget yourself, let Qi from the universe flow through you instead of giving away your own and will help your intentions toward your patients be clear and pure.

Note: I have the best response when I use 2 fingers (index and 2nd finger) and thumb. I have more control this way, but it is important for you to work with it and figure out what works for you.

Do the needle manipulations below until the Qi sensation is felt, then stop, though sometimes you want a stronger sensation than you are currently getting so you keep it up for a bit. You can also come back during the treatment and manipulate again to strengthen sensation. Many practitioners will manipulate on some points but not all and no one does all of these in one treatment. You pick the ones that work best for you and use them judiciously. That will come in time.

Are there more ways to manipulate than this? Absolutely. Some are stronger, some milder. But these are the most heavily tested, so you need to be familiar with them. The lifting and thrusting and rotating techniques are considered fundamental, while the others are more auxiliary methods.

Manipulation method	Discussion
Lifting and thrusting	This and the following Rotating method are the two most common. In this method you lift and insert repeatedly, inserting and withdrawing to the same depth, without actually removing the needle above the surface of the skin. You follow the needle rather than forcing it. You can manipulate with either a small range of motion (tonification) or a large range of motion (reduction or tonification in a big muscle with a larger range of Qi depth), but do not change the angle of insertion. (See Chapter 10 for methods.) I know of many practitioners who synchronize this with their breath.
Rotating	The 2nd of the two most common techniques. First, insert to depth. Then rotate the needle in the hole without changing the angle. When inserting perpendicularly, you can roll the needle back and forth between the pad of your thumb and the pad of your forefinger. Do not bend the needle. When you are inserting on an angle, rest the bottom of the needle on the 2nd joint of your index finger and roll it between the edge of this joint and the pad of your thumb.
Pressing	In the pressing method, insert needle to the proper depth. Press or tap around the base of the needle to "call" the Qi. You can press 'behind' the needle to block the Qi from going where you don't want it to go. You can also press, tap, or rub lightly along the line of the channel or along the path to guide the Qi where you want it to go. Regardless of channel direction, press where you want to direct the Qi.
Plucking	After inserting the needle to the proper depth,

Manipulation method	Discussion
	flick the handle of the needle with your index finger parallel to the direction you want the qi to go. More like thumping, actually. Alternately, you can just flick it to make the needle wiggle and call the qi. But be careful not to flick upward or the needle can come flying out!
Scraping	You need a coiled or rough handle on your needle to make this work. After the needle is inserted at the proper angle and to the proper depth, scrape either up or down on the handle with your fingernail, depending on what you want the Qi to do in order to make a vibration within. Don't bend the needle!
Shaking	This is a very gentle motion. All of them are, actually. This is like the motion of a pendulum with a small range. You can also "stir," even stirring the needle right out of the skin as a reducing technique to reduce excesses. Again, be aware of the whole needle, especially the tip of it when you do this.
Flying needle	Use this method only in areas where the needle is near or in large muscle. This is a strong stimulation. Once the needle is inserted to depth at the proper angle, spin it forward 180 degrees, then back about 90 degrees. Next make a hard rolling motion to make the needle spin in the hole. You can also spin it backwards the other direction. It's similar to the idea of spinning a top.
Trembling	This is a wiggling or trembling motion. Do tiny rotations of about 30 degrees while visualizing or imagining lifting or thrusting....without actually doing that.
Rotate and lift/thrust	This is a combination move of the two most

Manipulation method	Discussion
	common needle manipulations. Lift and thrust *while* rotating the needle.

NEEDLE RETENTION

How long do you keep those needles in the patient? Ancient texts say 28 minutes, but sometimes it depends on the environment you are treating in. Some practitioners keep the needles in 15-20 minutes, have the patient turn over and needle the other side for an additional 15-20. This varies, as there are different retentions for different applications.

Here are some rules of thumb.

Table 4.25	
Short duration	☯ Exterior problem and/or acute conditions (except for acute pain. See below) ☯ Sensitive patients
Longer duration	☯ Acute pain – longer lasting effects ☯ Interior problem and/or chronic problems.
Insert, get sensation, withdraw	☯ Small children ☯ Extremely sensitive patients ☯ Areas around the throat and eye ☯ Certain diseases such as frequent urination and diarrhea as examples.

Always be aware of your patient's condition, their state of mind/spirit, and the diseases with which they present. As an example, patients who have frequent urination or diarrhea might not appreciate your dogmatic "must leave the needles in for X minutes regardless!" approach.

During the patient's treatment, check in with them to see how Qi sensation is going. If they are no longer feeling it (which is super common), feel free to re-manipulate the salient points.

CHAPTER 10
Reinforcing and Reducing Methods

Reinforcing is also called tonification. Reinforcing methods in acupuncture are used to tonify deficiency (xu). Reducing methods are used to sedate, clear, or reduce excess (shi). You know which to use by doing using your diagnostic skills to arrive at a diagnosis and differentiation.[9] You use the techniques discussed in this chapter after the needle has been inserted and brought up the Qi sensations as discussed in this section.

You only reduce or reinforce at a *single* point, not both, though you can certainly reduce at one point and reinforce at another, using a variety of techniques on a single patient.

WHEN TO REDUCE, WHEN TO TONIFY

You reduce when pathogens, viruses, bacterium, exterior evils and so forth are too much. Often these exist in the body, becoming excessive when they cause illness, problems, or other forms of disharmony which lead to an imbalanced diseased state.

As an example, one might experience a damp invasion after hiking in a damp environment, prompting sensations of heaviness and coldness, brain fog, and maybe a headache that feels like a tight band around the head. Your job in such a case would be to use reducing methods to alleviate the excess damp in the body, balance the conditions within, and alleviate the patient's discomfort as a result.

---

[9] Calhoun, Diagnostic Skills in Chinese Medicine Book 1, ISBN 1096340577

The term "retention" expresses the same concept as the term excess. Phlegm retention caused by a diet of animal and dairy products with sugar and simple carbohydrate chasers.

I worked at Wendy's right after I got out of high school, a hamburger restaurant chain in the United States. I know. I didn't know any better. I saw people order hamburgers, fries and a soft drink then chase it down with a thick chocolate shake type drink afterwards. There was a lot of throat clearing and nose blowing in the parking lot after people ate because these types of foods cause inflammation and phlegm build up in the body due to the sugars, heavy greasy elements of the food, and dairy – phlegm retention.

Phlegm retention is a sensation you can feel in the throat and respiratory passages, but it might also express as foggy mind, masses (long term, lots of phlegm retention), and more. Blood stagnation is another example of retention you might treat with reducing methods. Blood should flow freely, can be retained in the body in the form of stagnation.

As a practitioner, you can sometimes feel deficiencies or excesses in the patient's body when you needle. You may detect an empty feeling – soft or hollow – which signals a deficiency. Or you may detect a tight feeling at depth or shallower signaling an excess or retention.

There are some factors to consider then using reducing/sedating techniques.

Consider:	Brief discussion
Condition of the body	Most acupuncture points have a dual regulating function, able to both tonify and reduce, depending on what the body needs.
	Stomach 36, for instance, could be sedated/reduced to decrease the activity of the stomach to treat

Consider:	Brief discussion
	stomach spasms or stomach pain. You can also tonify this point to promote digestion and alleviate food retention s/sx. This regulation is automatic, but you can enhance it with acupuncture methods. Another example is finger numbness, which you determine is due to Blood xu (deficiency). You could needle locally to increase the blood flow to the fingers, but in another condition (such as hypersensitivity in the fingers), you could use reducing techniques.
Function of the point	Though the vast majority of points are dually regulating, some have a leaning toward reduction or tonification. Some examples from just the Stomach channel: • Stomach 36 tonifies more readily than it reduces. • Stomach 40 reduces more readily than it tonifies and is often used to alleviate phlegm retention. • Stomach 34, the xi cleft point on the Stomach meridian, is prone to reduction, often used to stop acute pain related to the Stomach organ or channel.
Technique	For best treatment results, use tonifying techniques with points that are more prone to tonify the body. When you pick at reducing point, use reduction methods. In this way you are working *with* the natural leaning of the body and points instead of against these factors.

NEEDLE MANIPULATION +
REDUCTION AND TONIFICATION METHODS

Let's take the two predominant methods of needle manipulation, lifting and thrusting and needle rotation, to the next level. Let's combine them with reducing and tonifying methods to get the best response possible. This assumes you have inserted the needle in the right location and to the proper depth and have gotten the Qi sensation at the point.

How long do you use these techniques during a treatment?

That depends on the sensation. Usually, you do this less than 1 minute, stop, retain the needle a while (5 minutes or so), come back and stimulate again.

Using lifting and thrusting for reduction and tonification

Using the lifting and thrusting technique, you can push Qi into the point or draw out excesses. Points that have a Qi at a shallow depth will only require a small range of motion to get the sedation or tonification effect. Deeper locations and more muscular locations might have a greater range of motion or the same effect.

Tonification

You are using the needle in this setting to push more Qi into the point you are manipulation in order to tonify the point and thus the body. Make the whole needle an extension of your hand and visualize/imagine feeling the tip of the needle and see the Qi flowing into the point through the tip.

To use lifting and thrusting in order to tonify:
- ☯ On the push (thrust), push a little more forcefully than on the lifting motion. Push inward heavily without hurting your patient.

- ☯ Pause for a moment so that you don't "bounce." This also gives the Qi a chance to fill the point.

☯ Lift more gently so that you don't drag the Qi back with the needle.

Reduction

This is basically the opposite of the tonification method. You are using the tip of the needle to fish out excesses, pathogens, icky stuff that is being retained, etc.

To use lifting and thrusting in order to reduce:

☯ Push in gently, as if you are laying something very gently on a body of water without making a ripple. This assures that you are not introducing *more* of anything into this already excessive situation.

☯ Pause so that you don't bounce.

☯ Withdraw more forcefully, visualizing the excess being withdrawn from the site.

Using needle rotation for reduction and tonification

There are two methods for this. We'll talk about reduction and tonification in each of the methods below.

Method 1

This method has to do with the speed of the rotation – fast or slow – and with an even force and speed in both directions. The *median* speed of needle rotation is 1 to 2 times per second, rotating back and forth with the same speed to get the Qi sensation. To tonify or reduce, you can modify the speed as follows.

Tonification	To tonify, use a slower and gentler force to your rotations. This rotation is slower than the 1-2 times per second. My professor, Dr. Qiu, likened it to a gentle rain that falls slowly enough to nourish the soil.

Reduction	To reduce an excess condition, use a faster and more forceful rotation, faster than 1-2 times per second. This is more like a hard and fast rain that washes away before it can soak in, carrying the excess with it.

Method 2

While Method 1 uses an even speed for both tonification and reduction, this method changes in both speed and force, depending on which action you are performing.

The gentle part is like a slow recoil which has no impact on the Qi. It is similar in feel to a soft step or tiptoe that makes no sound.

Tonification or reinforcement	Rotate forward with thumb thrusting out from hand – rapidly and more forcefully. This is the tonification part of the manipulation. When you pull the thumb back toward you (the recoil), do so slowly and gently. Regardless of whether you are using your right hand or your left hand, when the thumb is out and away from the hand, this is yang and reinforcing. Pulling the thumb back toward the hand is more yin and reducing. This is why you pull the thumb back so gently.
Reduction	To reduce, simply reverse the above procedure. Pull your thumb back toward the hand more forcefully and faster to reduce, push the thumb forward slowly and gently.

Using respiration to reinforce or reduce
Synchronize your actions with your breath.

Many needling instructors will teach you to use breathing to further emphasize the action you want. To do this, start by getting the patient to regulate their breath. You can breath along with them to help them out if they don't know how. Synchronize your breath with theirs so that you are breathing together. You may have to teach them to breath long and slow breaths – a lot of us live our lives breathing shallowly and have no clue how to do this.

Reduction or Sedation	• Insert or manipulation on the *inhalation* This symbolically allows you to pull excess Qi out of the body through the tip of the needle, as if you are using suction to drain out the excess.* • Withdraw on the *exhalation.* Release that unwanted noise out of your body as you withdraw the needle.
Tonification or Reinforcing	• Insert/thrust or manipulate on the *exhale.* • Withdraw the needle on the *inhale.*

*It's important to have clear boundaries and to regulate breath, mind, and body so that you don't pull that Qi into your body. You want to let that excess flow through you without getting attached to you - release that to the universe where it belongs!

You can combine breath techniques with any of the other reduction and reinforcement techniques to "boost the signal," if you will.

Using needle direction to reinforce or reduce

Reinforcing	Aim the tip of the needle along the natural flow of the channel.
	In the Lung meridian, for instance, Qi naturally

	moves from the chest distally toward the tip of the thumb along the medial aspect of the arm. To reinforcing using the direction of the needle, you would aim the tip of the needle distally along the path of the channel.
Reducing	The opposite – aim the tip of the needle *against* the natural directional flow of the meridian. Using the Lung channel as an example again, the tip of the needle would be pointing toward the chest and in line with the path of the Lung meridian. This slows or partially blocks the Qi flow, which is great when you need to reduce and calm things down.

Qi movement can be different over the meridian's course. Keeping with our Lung meridian example, Qi in this channel flows downward from the chest along the medial aspect of the arm toward the thumb. But in the chest area it also flows upward because of Lung's dispersing function, which requires it to flow in all directions.

Qi goes both ways, in other words. Think about how you are trying to get the Qi to move. Do you want to send Qi to the desired area or block it?

Opening and closing the hold for reduction or tonification

This is pretty short and sweet. Your intent here plays a huge part – in this. Where the mind or intent goes, the Qi follows.

Reduction	Leave the hole open to allow pathogenic influences to escape. Combine this with other reduction methods for greatest effect.

	You can lift forcefully to siphon off excess, retain the needle, stimulate again, then leave the hole open when the needle is removed.
Tonification	Close the hole to retain Qi within the body. Again, combine this with other tonification/reinforcing methods for best effect. As an example, push Qi in with forceful thrust or rotation. When you remove the needle, remove gently then quickly press the hole closed. The most important point here is to have the intent to retain the Qi when you close the hole!

THE EVEN METHOD

Some disorders are atypical of deficiency or excess. Conditions like overuse could be a good example of this.

Let's say you get a new apartment, but hate the color. You get some paint and paint rollers and you get busy. You spend many hours rolling the paint on the top of the wall and even on the ceiling. The next day, your shoulders, unaccustomed to these particular repetitive motions are sore and achy and you are more than a little miserable.

This isn't a true excess or deficiency, but it's still pretty uncomfortable. You go to acupuncture for some relief and she or he says you have a blockage in your Qi and Blood flow to the area, which is causing the discomfort. Your acupuncturist might use and even method to get things moving in the area. That would look like this:

1. Your acupuncturist inserts a needle into the right point to focus on this problem – maybe Small Intestine 14 is the point where it seems to be really knotted. She or he

inserts to the proper depth, then gets the Qi sensation.

2. Said acupuncturist then rotates the needle evenly and gently at a moderate speed to bring a mild sensation to the area.

3. The needle is withdrawn at a moderate speed.

It is the intent that determines this more than the technique.

Another good use for this method is for encouraging better blood flow. I've had colleague do this for me when I need to go in for blood work. My blood seems to flow slowly and it's hard to find my vessels at the elbow, so I generally end up with a butterfly needle in the back of my hand. Using an even method like this makes it easier for the phlebotomist to hit the vessel on the first stick and the blood flows more easily.

SECTION 3
Precautions, Contraindications & Management of Accidents

This fleshes out a little more detail about practical clinical approaches to what to do when an accident occurs as well as preventing them in the first place by understanding the precautions and contraindications around acupuncture.

This page intentionally left blank.

CHAPTER 11
Precautions and Contraindications

Precautions are a yield sign in acupuncture. You could do these things and use these points, but you have to be very judicious. Contraindications are a hard stop. You just don't do these things and with good reason. This chapter explores both of those things.

CONTRAINDICATIONS

There are just some points that shouldn't been needled and there are some situations that also have contraindications.

Contraindication	Discussion
Points that aren't needled	• Stomach 17 This point is on the nipple. We don't needle that. Like ever. • Ren 8 This point is the center of the umbilicus. It is purely a reference point for locating other acupuncture points on the abdomen and lower abdomen. You never needle it. Ren 8 is connected with Mother Earth and with the universe, so it can regulate the function of the whole body. You *can* use indirect moxa (moxa on ginger or salt) at Ren 8, you can cup it (which looks *so* weird), and you can apply herbal therapies here. But never needle it.
Site of wounds, ulcers and scars	We don't needle *into* these areas. We do sometimes needle around the edges. Scar tissue can be treated very effectively by needling around the edge, actually. I've also treated shingles outbreaks by using a plum blossom

Contraindication	Discussion
	needle to release heat around the outside edge of the lesions. Works quite well.
Infants	Never needle the vertex of the head when the fontanel is not closed! You can see the pulsation here when the fontanels have not closed over. You *can* do acupuncture on infants, though acupressure, tuina, and non-inserting methods such as Japanese acupuncture are more appropriate for infants. Their skin is so tender, and the Qi is so superficial that you can stimulate the skin and affect the whole body. Any acupuncture for infants has a very low needle retention time.
Pregnant women	There are points that are expressly forbidden for pregnant patients, as they are too strong and disturb the fetus, or are too descending and could jump start labor inappropriately. Some of these points *are* used *during* the birthing time to help promote smooth and efficient labor. If you start looking for contraindicated points for pregnant patients in Chinese medical literature and online you will find they don't always agree. As a rule, however, these are what you can't needle during pregnancy and fetal development: • Large Intestine 4 • Spleen 6 • Bladder 60 • Bladder 67 • Gallbladder 21 This point has a strong descending function that is great in labor, not so great during pregnancy when the mother wants the baby developing well. There are also pregnancy contraindications regarding the stage of fetal development:

Contraindication	Discussion
	• First trimester (1st 3 months) Do not needle points on the lower abdomen or lumbosacral region. This is where the baby is developing and could stir too much Qi, disturbing the fetus. • Second and third trimesters Points on the upper *and* lower abdomen and lumbosacral region. As the baby gets larger in the womb and the fundus expands, the baby is also developing higher and higher in the mother's body. The same thing applies as before – stirring too much Qi by using points in this region could disturb the fetus.

Conditions in which acupuncture is contraindicated	• After severe bleeding, diarrhea, or sweating
	Like after childbirth (bleeding) or conditions of shock or of extreme exercise in which there is heavy sweating (which reduces the yin, body fluids, and qi – acupuncture has a reducing/sedating effect at this point).
	
	The body is under stress and trying to regulate in these conditions. If you are needling for a sports injury, make sure the patient is adequately hydrated!
	
	• Severe xu (deficiency)
	Same reasons and conditions are present as above. The body cannot adjust to or handle Qi stimulation in this case.
	
	• Temporary conditions in which acupuncture is contraindicated:
	   o Drunk patients
	     Alcohol in the body causes a disording of Qi. You don't think it will happen, but it very well could. I

Contraindication	Discussion
	treated a functioning alcoholic for some time that occasionally lapsed and came in drunk.
	o Extreme anger or fright This also deregulates the Qi, causing it to rush upward.
	o Extremely hungry, full, or thirsty You need a balance of these extremes. Fullness causes discomfort and rebellion of Stomach Qi. Emptiness of either food or drink causes weakened state.
	o Too tired, overworked, etc. Same as hungry/full/thirsty but with energy rather than physically consumable substances.
	• Patients that bleed very easily Examples would include hemophiliacs or those on strong blood thinners. This is why you need a good patient intake, history (including pharmaceuticals taken) and consent forms! If you patient is taking maintenance dose blood thinners and understands the bruising and bleeding risks, then you can treat that patient.
	• Pregnant women with a history of miscarriage.

Points that require caution include:

Caution required	More information
Points near nerve trunks, large blood vessels, tendons	You *can* needle these points, but do not do strong manipulations or manipulations with large amplitude.
Points near organs	No deep insertions at these points. Some examples are Gallbladder 21 at the top of the shoulder. The apex of the lung in some patients can come up quite close to the surface in some patients. Deep perpendicular insertion here is expressly forbidden for this reason. Even with an oblique insertion, do not do manipulations of large amplitude here. The same would be true in the upper back and chest, over the kidneys, bladder,etc.

Additionally, there are different stimulation intensities for different body constitutions and disease conditions.

Intensity of Manipulation

Different conditions need different intensities of manipulation and stimulation.

Often you see the reaction to the manipulation with the tenting of the skin and with surface reddening. Not all patients react this way, however. Some might react more deeply in the body where it is hidden from your eyes.

For this effect:	Use these:
Strong	• Thick needles • Long needles • Deep insertion • Big amplitude in manipulation • Frequent manipulations

For this effect:	Use these:
	• Longer retention time
Mild	• Thin needle • Shorter needle • Shallow insertion • Small manipulation amplitude • Less frequent manipulation • Shorter retention time

Use different intensities for different constitutions and body types.

Constitution or type	Appropriate stimulation level
Weak constitution	Milder stimulation.
Strong constitution	Stronger stimulation
Yang body type	Milder stimulation People with Yang constitutions have fast moving Qi and tend to be more needle sensitive.
Yin body type	Stronger stimulation Qi moves more slowly for these folks, so they are less needle sensitive.

You also use different methods depending on different disease patterns. Consider these:

Pattern	Appropriate stimulation level
Exterior condition	Shallow insertion. You don't want to drive the pathogen deeper into the body with a deep insertion!
Interior condition	Use a deeper insertion and retain the needles longer. It takes the body longer to adjust when an interior condition is present.
Xu (deficiency) state	Use tonification methods. You won't know if you need a milder or stronger stimulation until you assess the

Pattern	Appropriate stimulation level
	patient.
Shi (excess) states	Use reducing methods. You won't know if you need a milder or stronger stimulation until you assess the patient.
Cold conditions	Cold can be a shi cold or a xu cold. Deep insertion, longer retention. The concern is that qi will not be able to move freely. Qi also recedes further into the body as winter progresses. You may have to call it up as it takes time for it to come out of "hibernation" in the winter.
Heat	Can be a shi heat or a xu heat. In general, use a shallow insertion and shorter duration.

This page intentionally left blank.

Acupuncture Techniques 101 - Chapter 11

CHAPTER 12
Managing Accidents

Sometimes no matter how careful you are or how much you work to prevent accidents, stuff happens. This chapter covers what to do and how you might prevent the most common accidents in an acupuncture clinic.

ACU-SHOCK

Acu-shock is pretty much just what it sounds like – shock induced by acupuncture. Signs and symptoms look like this:

Severity	S/sx
Mild	• Weakness • Dizziness • Vertigo • Cold sweats • Palpitations • Shortness of breath • Feeling of oppression in the chest • Nausea • Pallor • Weak pulse
Severe	• Cold extremities • Cyanosis of the lips and/or nails • Drop in blood pressure • Incontinence of urine or stool • Loss of consciousness

Acu-shock can have a number of causative factors. I list them below along with what you can do to prevent this:

- Nervous tension

  Extremely nervous patients are more susceptible to acu-shock. To prevent this, you need to be able to relax and calm the patient before you treat them. Patients who have never had acupuncture before, for example, might have a lot of questions or fears.

I spend time talking with them about what is going to happen and how it's going to feel, how the most sensitive areas are mostly on the hands and feet, I teach them to breath with me to promote more calm, insert a needle into my own forearm to show how much it really doesn't hurt, etc. Even if I don't get more than a few needles in for treatment, this is better than acu-shock and the patient appreciates it.

For new patients, you might try fewer points and mild manipulation. Watch them closely for their reaction.

☯ Delicate constitution, hunger, fatigue, extreme weakness after severe diarrhea, bleeding or sweating
All of these cause a drop in Qi. Make sure your patients are properly hydrated, fed, rested, etc. Many practitioners even put instructions to eat lightly and stay hydrated before an appoitment in their online write-ups and clinic forms.

☯ Improper patient positioning
Put patients in a position that is comfortable for them. I've had back pain patients that couldn't manage any position other than lateral recumbent. Work with them. If you have a massage chair this can be good for that patient population.

☯ Manipulation that is too forceful
Communicate with your patient during the treatment and watch them after the needles are in.

☯ Treatment environment that is too hot or too cold
Monitor your patients, check in on them during the

treatment while the needles are in and they are resting. Makes sure nothing needs to be changed or adjusted.

Treatment of acu-shock

And sometimes, no matter what you do or how careful you are, it happens. Here's how you handle it if it does.

Most cases:

- ☯ Stop needling immediately and remove all needles
- ☯ Help the patient lie down with head lower, feet elevated, clothes loosened
- ☯ Offer patient sweet or warm water

For severe cases:

- ☯ Do acu*pressure* at the following sites. These are actually pretty great points for many syncope events. (Some texts say acupuncture, but....really? That's what got us here in the first place. I'm betting patient confidence is low right now. No more needles.)

Point	Brief info
Du 24	Opens the sensory orifices, nice point for fainting and feeling like you are about to. This on the philtrum under the nose. If you divided this into 1/3's, this would be the dividing line between the top 1/3 and the bottom 2/3.
Du 25	Right at the tip of the nose. We never needle it because who wants to get punched by a patient? It's one of those contraindicated points. But you can pinch it with medium pressure and open the Du channel, which goes right through the center of the body. That'll wake you up!
LI 4	This points moves a tremendous amount of

Point	Brief info
	Qi. Press the point against the second metacarpal bone for a stronger stimulation.
PC 6	This point is 2 cun proximal to the medial crease at the wrist and right in between the two tendons you see when this point is facing you and you make a fist. PC 6 is a great point for nausea, vomiting, motion sickness, and Qi rebelling upwards.
St 36	Stomach 36 is below the knee and, so said my energetic professor – for like 4 full lectures - is the most important point on the body. You'll spend a lot of time learning about why this is so and what all it can do. Think of it as the pivot around which your own personal solar system spins. It's that important. Great for fainting with symptoms of coldness – like cold sweats, feeling cold, as well as woozy and about to pass out.
Kd 1	Press with your thumb or with a massage tool to stimulate the adrenal glands. This point is on the bottom of the foot and right on the center-line if you divide the foot down the middle from toes to heel. Now curl your toes down like you are trying to touch your heel with your big toe. See that divot just below the ball of your foot and in the center? That's Kidney 1. Take a peek at your Deadman book. A picture is worth a thousand words.
PC 9	This regulates the heart function and improves blood flow. It's located right at the tip of your middle finger. That's right, the one you gesticulate

Point	Brief info
	with in traffic. And stop aiming your Pericardium channel at people. Keep that energy inside where it belongs.
Du 20	At the very top of the head, Du 20 lifts the Qi up to the head and clears the fog that closes in on people who feel like they are losing consciousness. Some texts recommend moxa, which will work, but if you're already nervous about the acu-shock, do you really want to set their hair on fire? I'd go for acupressure. But the answer is probably "moxa" on a test.
Ren 4	This point tonifies the Yuan Qi. Use moxa to warm and tonify the body here.
Ren 6	This is the "ocean of Qi" – the Dantian, the center of gravity. Use moxa here to warm and tonify and bring the person back to center.
Ren 8	In the center of the umbilicus. Use a salt cake or ginger here with a moxa cone to tonify and warm the body.

☯ If it's really an emergency, like the patient has lost consciousness and you can't stop it, call 911. Don't spend a lot of time evaluating. Better to be safe than sorry.

I've had this happen a couple of times. Both times the patient let me know they were feeling weird and getting a bit sweaty. I pulled the needles and did acupressure and moxa both times and all was well. The patient felt better and was fine afterwards too. And in both cases the problem was poor nutrition – neither had eaten since the day before. Your mileage may vary.

Sometimes you come back to remove the needles and find you can't get one out. The Qi and/or the fiber around the needle grabs it and won't let go. Sometimes you can't even manipulate it. This is a stuck needle. There are a couple of reasons this happens.

Hint: Use fewer needles, use points without strong stimulation, manipulate very gently for new patients and you'll see less of all of these acupuncture accidents!

Reason	Discussion
Nervousness of patient and/or strong spasm of local muscle	Can get stuck because the patient is tense or nervous and can't relax, causing a spasm in the local area. Can also happen at insertion – strong stimulation with either manual manipulation or electro-stimulation, causing muscle to move. This happens more often where there are more tendons, like near a joint or near the eyebrow where the muscles are already tight. **What to do:** • Ask pt to relax. This is key for any of these actually. You want patient to relax their whole body, which will relax the stuck spot as well. Breathing exercises will help. • Leave the needle in place a little while longer. It may just not be done at the point. Try removing it again after you remove the others. • Massage or tap gently around the point. This can distribute the Qi and release the muscle. • Insert another needle nearby – same deal. Draws the Qi away and weakens the spasm.

Reason	Discussion
	Don't needle too far away – you want it pretty close by so the same muscle or muscle group to start multi tasking and releases that stuck needle.
Rotating the needle with a large amplitude or in only one direction.	This twists the fibers around the tip of the needle and tangles it up somewhat. **What to do:** Rotate the needle in the opposite direction. You might not remember which direction you went originally…try a very small range of rotation one direction or the other to see what works better. Always move the needle back and forth when you manipulate! Even with the flying technique you rotate the needle back then fly other direction.
Patient changed position	Some patients don't move during treatment at all because they are terrified to move, which can cause stuck needles due to tension. Some patients are wiggly and gesticulate a lot with hands and this too will cause stuck needle – they've moved the muscle, the muscle starts grabbing the needle. Patients also fall asleep and move around without knowing it. Finally, it could have been you – like you moved an arm thinking it was better and the muscle reacted. Usually no big deal. **What to do:** Put them back in the original position. Make this quite passive. Instruct them to relax the affected body part while you gently move it back in place. This will often relax the muscle. If not, use the suggestions above about tapping and inserting another needle.

BENT NEEDLES

You go back to take needles out and one is bent! Or you hear the patient yell for you, go in and this has happened.

It's blissfully rare for this to happen. . . unless you're a physical therapist or chiropractor practicing "IMS" (intra-muscular stimulation) or "DN" (dry needling). They seem to think that's common and normal. IMS and DN, is acu-geek code by the way. In our language it means "people practicing acupuncture without a license or proper training and calling it something different so they can skirt the scope of practice laws." If you want to see a bunch of acupuncturists lose their collective mind, mention this in a room full of them.

Causes of bent needles

Cause	Discussion
Unskillful or too forceful manipulation	This can cause the needle to strike hard tissue (bone, tendon or other resistant tissue). Too much force and not following the needle can cause that too. Then you are working at cross purposes with the needle. Have the intention to follow the path of the needle and not force. Pretend it is a stiff thread you're trying not to bend.
Needling in a tight area	If you are on a point that is very close to a bone or tendon bent needles are more likely.
Posture change	If the patient changes their posture a needle can bend. As an example, when I needle on the lateral side of the lower leg I prop the foot and lower leg up before I do so because I know that when people are on the table in a supine position that their feet will tend to roll outward when they fall asleep or relax. That can put pressure on the needle and cause it to bend. You can't control sudden jerks and repositionings when people fall asleep, though.

Cause	Discussion
Collision of needle from external force	That can be the foot flop I just mentioned or the sudden jerk or position change. It can also be from a blanket you cover your patient with.

I use really light polar fleece blankets to cover people. I also have some yoga blocks I put between people's feet and sometimes next to their elbows to lift the blanket up off of the needles. I generally set up a heat lamp over their feet to help keep them warm too.

Also, watch where your body is in relation to the needles when you are inserting. It's easy to get lost in the task and forget you are leaning against the needle. |
| Improper management of stuck needles | Applying too much force to remove a stuck needle can cause a spasm that bends it. And sometimes that stuck needle is stuck because it's bent. |

What to do about bent needles:
Don't manipulate the needle at all and don't try to withdraw it forcefully. Put the patient back into the original position you needled them in and do this passively – have them relax the limb and you move it. Follow the course of the needle and slowly withdraw it.

BROKEN NEEDLES

Everybody has a work nightmare or two. This is one of mine. It's never happened, but I still fear it. This is when a needle breaks off at or below the surface of the skin.

The most common reason for a needle to break is fatigue from re-use and sterilization (so what am I worried about? I use disposable single-use!). The most common site of breakage is where the shaft meets the handle. Very thin needles are more susceptible (both re-usable and single use), as are poor quality needles. Be aware that even with care and single use needles, strong e-stim can cause needle breakage. Use a hefty needle instead of thin needles for e-stim.

To prevent this kind of thing to the best of your ability:
- Use quality needles
- Look at your needles before you insert.
- If you use re-usable needles, inspect them carefully after sterilization. Use a clean cotton ball to test the needle for burs and rough spots that might indicate wear.
- *Never* insert a needle all the way to the handle!
- Use an appropriately thick gauge single use needle for e-stim.

Something you can't control are very strong muscle spasms that break the needle as opposed to merely bending it.

What to do about it if it should happen on your watch:
- Keep the patient calm. Don't change their posture at all or the needle could go in deeper.
- If the end of the broken part of the needle is exposed above the surface of the skin, remove it with our fingers or with hemostats/foreceps
- If the end of the needle is level with the skin, press very gently around the edge and remove the needle with foreceps if you can.
- If the broken part is *below* skin surface, call 911 so that the patient can be taken to a hospital for surgical procedures to remove the broken part. This is beyond our legal scope of practice in the United States as a licensed acupuncturist.

HEMATOMA

After withdrawal of the needle, you might see bleeding and bruising, maybe with local swelling and possible limited movement. Hematomas form as a result of subcutaneous bleedout. This can happen when circulation is poor, if a patient is hemophiliac, has poor Spleen Qi function, or is on blood thinners. Older patients are also more likely to have this happen.

If you see blood drops after you withdraw, immediately press on it to see if you can stop bleeding. If it's mild, it should respond quickly. If it's an artery, will be worse.

Usually these bruises are small and they are no big deal to the patient. If a large-ish hematoma forms, have the patient apply a cool compress during the first 24 hours, then afterwards use warm compress or moxa to warm the area and start clearing the blood out. You can also use herbs to stop bleeding and massage after the bruise forms to help blood reabsorb into body.

Prevention:
- Aging patients and those who tend to bruise easily. Use mild stimulation and thinner gauge needles. Think about Japanese acupuncture – they use very very shallow needling to good effect.

- Be one with the needle, grasshopper. Train yourself to extend your Qi and sensations down the needle to the tip, similar to what fencers do when they sword fight.

  When you hit a blood vessel you will feel a tight sensation. If you keep pushing it will suddenly feel empty. If you feel that, remove the needle and press with a cotton ball because you just hit a vessel.

  That said, you can also feel a similar tight sensation when you are in muscular areas. If muscles feel very tight, this could be an excess.

Points by the spine and neck are also very tight, due to the tendinous connections that run between the bones. I mention this because Gallbladder 20 is such a common point to use for neck pain and for headaches. There is a big artery and a huge nerve bundle close to this. Your points location instructor will teach you what needle angles to use to avoid bleeding here.

POST NEEDLING SENSATIONS

Sensations in the general body and around the needling sites *can* follow a treatment by a few minutes to a day or more.

Localized sensations
The more common sensation is a localized sensations where the needles were located. This might be a soreness or a buzz. Massage at the site helps with both.

Generalized sensations
This is a feeling of low energy or can be felt as poor sleep. This is relatively common when the patient gets too tired after a treatment or is chronically overworked. It can also be due to stimulation that was too strong during the treatment or because the needles were retained too long causing a Qi depletion.

Let's revisit that "too tired after treatment" thing. I've had patients tell me they got a burst of energy after a treatment, went and got a bunch of things done, then didn't sleep well after that. That's what I'm talking about. I've even done this myself. You can warn patients about this, but you can't keep them from doing it.

PREVENTING INJURY TO ORGANS

That's a pretty huge priority. Let's look at individual organs and how not to injure them. If you do accidentally puncture an organ or any of the 'danger' tissues below, call 911. Then call your lawyer.

Organ	Prevention of injury
Lung	A lung puncture is a pneumothorax. This occurs when the lung is punctured by a needle and begins to collapse the alveoli. These tend to cause a cascading collapse. The patient feels nothing at first, then shortness of breath and cough. If the needle is still in, this causes bigger holes to tear in the lung tissue. S/sx: Chest tightness and pain as the alveoli collapse, cough, shortness of breath, palpitations. If severe, dyspnea, pallor, cyanosis, cold sweats, drop in blood pressure, coma, death. Anytime you put a needle in the chest or upper back and between the intercostal spaces you are needling above the lung. The risk increases if your angle and depth or wrong or if you do strong manipulations. If you needle at the proper angle and depth, this should not be a problem. The points where this is most likely to occur are at Lu 1, Lu 2, St 12, all of the thorax points on the Stomach channel, Gb 21, and all intercostal spaces both front and back. When a needle goes too deep at these points it hits the pleura first. It is a soft feeling that the patient can feel but you probably can't. If this were to happen, remove the needles and keep the patient in a stable position. A reclining position rather than lying down makes it easier to breathe. Call 911.
Liver, heart, stomach, spleen	The liver is about the level of the 6th intercostal space and around the sternum on the right side of the trunk. Enlarged livers can pose more risk of danger. These will extend below the lower costal area even on the exhaled breath. The spleen is on the opposite side of the body but at a similar location. The stomach . . . well, you know where your stomach is. Patients will feel pain if an organ is punctured. Liver or spleen puncture causes abdominal pain, rigidity in the abdominal muscles and/or rebound pain with pressure.

Organ	Prevention of injury
	All of the points in the intercostal spaces on the lower costal areas (both front and back) are in the danger zone, including Stomach channel, Liver channel, and Gallbladder channel points on the trunk. Again, needling at the correct angle and insertion depth should keep you safe, though even Stomach 19 can be at risk for hitting an enlarged heart.
	If the heart is punctured the patient will feel a severe stabbing in the chest, a tearing pain, and will go into shock.
Kidney	When you are needling the back points in the T11-L3 areas, you are in the area where the Kidneys are. The Bladder channel points in this area are the most commonly needled. Never needle deeper than ½ to 1 cun in depth here, even less than that with thinner people.
	Kidney puncture will cause pain in the lumbar region, tenderness, and percussion pain around the kidney area. There can be blood in the urine, even a drop in blood pressure and coma.
Intestines and bladder	Any point on the anterior aspect of the trunk below the costal area could be susceptible to puncture. When a patient has a full bladder the risk of bladder puncture increases, so always have them go to the bathroom before you begin needling.
	The lower abdominal points on the Stomach, Spleen, Ren, and Kidney channel are the most likely areas where a bladder or intestinal puncture can occur.
Occipital area	The base of the skull has major blood vessels, the nerve root of the spinal cord, the brain stem, and the spinal cord to worry about. This can be a scary area to needle in, but has some great points that treat a lot of stuff.
	You will feel strong tight sensations here when you needle. If you needle more than 1 cun in depth here, hit a hard sensation, then break through it, you could be in real trouble, as you may have just punctured the spinal cord.
	Consider using ½ cun needles in this area. When you are needling near the base of the skull, like at Du 15 or Gb 20,

Organ	Prevention of injury
	don't insert perpendicularly and don't angle upward toward the brain. Ask you point locations instructor for help. If the brain is punctured mild s/sx include headache, nausea, vomiting. Severe s/sx include dyspnea, convulsions, coma, death. If the spinal cord is punctured, mild s/sx include an electric shock sensation that radiates to the end of the limbs. If it's severe, then paralysis of the extremities or limited movement as well as decreased sensation in the limbs.
Posterior midline	The Du channel is right along the posterior midline and the jiaji points are very close to this as well. The spinal cord runs through the middle of the spine, so *never* needle deeper than 0.8 cun.

To avoid puncturing organs, the spinal cord, and blood vessels, your very best prep is 1) being able to feel the Qi in the needle and regulate your own Qi and 2) intimately understanding and memorizing the underlying anatomical structures under the acupuncture points.

Also understand proper angles and depths for the points.

This page intentionally left blank.

ABOUT THE AUTHOR

Cat Calhoun is a licensed acupuncture practitioner in the State of Texas and soon to be in the State of Florida as well. She attended AOMA Graduate School of Integrative Medicine, earning a Masters degree in Acupuncture and Oriental Medicine. She is passionate about teaching, both formally and informally. Cat has single-handedly created and managed CatsTCMNotes.com since 2008, dispensing notes and clinical pearls to students and practitioners for the past 11 years. She is also passionate about learning, and is currently in love with Master Tung's Acupuncture system.

This book, *Acupuncture Techniques 101: Safety, CNT, and Needling Techniques*, has a companion book for the 2nd half of basic acupuncture techniques in Chinese medicine (needling styles, gua sha, cupping, etc.). Look for *Acupuncture Techniques 102: Cupping, Moxibustion, Gua sha, E-Stim, and More* on Amazon. This companion text covers the basics of cupping, cutaneous needle therapy, electro-acupuncture, gua sha, moxibustion, and bleeding techniques. Both of these books are vital for framing your understanding of the basic acupuncture treatment methods and safety, critical information you need in order to treat effectively in clinic. Both books are available in digital and print format.